Best of Sleep Apnea 2016
An Annual Collection of Scientific Literature

Teofilo Lee-Chiong MD
Somnologist

This is the problem – time (or rather not having enough of it.)

Our understanding of sleep medicine is changing each day, and the rate of growth in knowledge will only accelerate along with our inability to keep up with new research findings. It would take at least 12,540 minutes to read all the important published articles related to sleep disordered breathing in any given year. Twelve thousand minutes that could be used for other types of meaningful work and leisure.

This is a *personal* selection of articles that I believe will influence future medical management and research in sleep-disordered breathing. Selected from hundreds of journal articles in medical periodicals, this compendium consists of concise summaries of some of the finest scientific literature on sleep apnea published from October 2015 to December 2016.

I hope that you'll find this collection useful.

Teofilo Lee-Chiong MD
Professor of Medicine
School of Medicine
University of Colorado Denver

3

ISBN-13: 978-1544046563
ISBN-10: 1544046561

Contents

6MWD: six minute walk distance
AASM: American Academy of Sleep Medicine
AF: atrial fibrillation
AHI: apnea hypopnea index
AI: apnea index
ALS: amyotrophic lateral sclerosis
APAP: auto-adjusting positive airway pressure
ASV: adaptive servo ventilation
BMI: body mass index
BNP: pro-brain natriuretic peptide
BP: blood pressure
BPAP: bilevel positive airway pressure
BQ: Berlin questionnaire
CAD: coronary artery disease
CAI: central apnea index
CHF: congestive heart failure
CI: confidence interval
CKD: chronic kidney disease
CompSA: complex sleep apnea
COPD: chronic obstructive pulmonary disease
CPAP: continuous positive airway pressure
CRF: chronic respiratory failure
CRP: C reactive protein
CSA: central sleep apnea
CSR: Cheyne-Stokes respiration
CV: cardiovascular
DBP: diastolic blood pressure
DM: diabetes mellitus
EEG: electroencephalography
EF: ejection fraction
ESS: Epworth Sleepiness Scale
FEV_1: forced expiratory volume in 1 second
FOSQ: Functional Outcomes of Sleep Questionnaire
FVC: forced vital capacity
HF: heart failure
HI: hypopnea index
HR: heart rate

HST: home sleep testing
HTN: hypertension
ICER: incremental cost-effectiveness ratio
ICU: intensive care unit
IH: intermittent hypoxia
IL: interleukin
LTOT: long-term oxygen therapy
LV: left ventricle
LVEF: left ventricular ejection fraction
LVH: left ventricular hypertrophy
MAD: mandibular advancement device
MI: myocardial infarction
MRI: magnetic resonance imaging
MSNA: muscle sympathetic nerve activity
N1: stage N1 sleep
N2: stage N2 sleep
N3: stage N3 sleep
NIV: noninvasive ventilation
NPV: negative predictive value
NREM: non-rapid eye movement sleep
NYHA: New York Heart Association
O_2: oxygen
OA: oral appliance
OAHI: obstructive apnea hypopnea index
ODI: oxygen desaturation index
OHS: obesity hypoventilation syndrome
OSA: obstructive sleep apnea
$PaCO_2$: arterial PCO_2
PAP: positive airway pressure
$PetCO_2$: end-tidal PCO_2
PPV: positive predictive value
PSG: polysomnography
PSQI: Pittsburgh Sleep Quality Index
$PtcCO_2$: transcutaneous PCO_2
PVT: psychomotor vigilance test
QALY: quality-adjusted life-year
QOL: quality of life
RCT: randomized controlled trial
RDI: respiratory disturbance index

RERA: respiratory effort related arousal
RIP: respiratory inductance plethysmography
RLS: restless legs syndrome
RV: right ventricle
SaO$_2$: oxygen saturation
SaO$_2$min: minimum oxygen saturation
SBP: systolic blood pressure
SDB: sleep disordered breathing
SE: sleep efficiency
SOL: sleep onset latency
SOS: sultan of sleep
SWS: slow wave sleep
TIA: transient ischemic attack
TNFα: tumor necrosis factor alpha
TV: tidal volume
UA: upper airway

☐
Obstructive sleep apnea is not uncommon among patients complaining of insomnia or RLS symptoms. This cohort consisted of 1,900 adults who underwent PSG studies. Over 30% of patients with symptoms of insomnia or RLS, but no sleep apnea symptoms, were found to have OSA (AHI > 5).
Bianchi MT et al. Acta Neurol Scand. 2016 Jan;133(1):61-7.

☐
Sleep disordered breathing is present in nearly 4 of every 5 cardiac surgery patients. In the prospective NU-SLEEP study, no, mild, moderate and severe SDB were noted in 22.6%, 35.9%, 25.9% and 15.6% of 1,005 patients undergoing cardiac surgery, respectively. Postoperative AF occurred in 13.6%, 13.5%, 31.9% and 52.5% of patients with no, mild, moderate and severe SDB, respectively. Ejection fraction was lower, and levels of atrial and brain natriuretic peptides were higher in the severe SDB group compared to those with milder disease.
Sezai A et al. Int J Cardiol. 2017 Jan 15;227:342-346.

☐
There are significant ethnic differences in OSA prevalence among patients presenting with acute coronary syndrome. This article reported data from the ISAACC Trial and Sleep and Stent Study. Overnight sleep study was used to identify OSA (AHI ≥ 15) in 1,961 Brazilian, Burmese, Chinese, Indian, Malay and Spanish patients. Prevalence of OSA differed among the difference ethnicities (from highest to lowest): Spanish (63.1%), Chinese (50.2%), Malay (47.9%), Burmese (43.5%), Brazilian (41.2%) and Indian (36.1%) patients. The effect of BMI on OSA was most pronounced in the Chinese population.
Koo CY et al. Heart Lung Circ. 2016 Nov 15.

☐
Residence at high altitude increases the likelihood of OSA in patients with CV disease. This study recruited patients with CAD (n = 398), with AF (n = 144) and without CV disease (n = 292) who were living at sea level, moderate altitude or high altitude. Persons with CV disease living at high altitude had a higher risk for sleep apnea (determined by PSG) than those

living at lower altitudes, with highest risk seen in men who had CAD or AF.

Otero L et al. High Alt Med Biol. 2016 Dec;17(4):336-341.

☐

Seventy percent of adult bariatric surgery patients have OSA. In this prospective, multicenter trial, 71% of 197 consecutive patients who underwent overnight cardiorespiratory recording had OSA (90% of men and 60% of women). The OSA group had larger mean neck and waist circumference and higher BMI compared to the non-OSA group. The only inter-group difference in women was a larger neck circumference.

Peromaa-Haavisto P et al. Obes Surg. 2016 Jul;26(7):1384-90.

☐

Prevalence of OSA is high in individuals with serious mental illnesses. This meta-analysis of 2 articles reported that the prevalence of OSA (AHI > 5) was 25.7% in those with serious mental illness (clinical studies), including 36.3% in persons with major depressive disorder, 24.5% in bipolar disorder, and 15.4% in schizophrenia. In population cohort studies, the prevalence of OSA was 10.7% in persons with serious mental illness, and 19.8% in major depressive disorder. Increased prevalence of OSA was linked to increasing age and BMI.

Stubbs B et al. J Affect Disord. 2016 Jun;197:259-67.

☐

Truck drivers of dangerous goods have a high prevalence of OSA. This study also confirmed that the risk of NMAs was significantly increased in persons with untreated severe OSA. The prevalence of OSA (diagnosed by PSG) and the risk of MVAs and NMAs were assessed in 283 truck drivers of dangerous goods. Although none of the subjects reported having OSA-related symptoms before screening, 49.1% had suspected OSA based on the Sleep Disorder Score (SDS) questionnaire, and 35.7% had OSA during PSG. The frequency of MVAs and NMAs was determined at baseline in all drivers, and again after 2 years of CPAP therapy in subjects with severe OSA. There was a significant association between OSA severity and NMAs, with a near 5-fold increased risk of NMAs in the group with severe OSA. The rate of NMAs fell to the level seen in non-OSA drivers after 2 years of CPAP therapy.

Garbarino S et al. Sleep Med. 2016 Sep;25:98-104.

☐
Nearly 1 in 10 male Japanese public transportation drivers have OSA.
This study investigated the prevalence of OSA among 2,389 occupational
drivers. Subjects underwent HST. Polysomnography and MSLT were
performed if the AHI was ≥ 15 on HST. Prevalence of OSA was 9.8% in this
population.
Sasai-Sakuma T et al. J Occup Environ Med. 2016 May;58(5):455-8.

☐
Poor sleep quality is common among athletes in team sports. In this
report involving 175 highly trained rugby and cricket athletes, mean
nightly sleep duration was 7.9 ± 1.3 hours. Many athletes were poor
sleepers (50%), had significant daytime sleepiness (28%), snored (38%) or
reported witnessed apneas (8%).
Swinbourne R et al. Eur J Sport Sci. 2016 Oct;16(7):850-8.

☐
**An estimated 8% of college football players are believed to suffer from
SDB.** Investigators, suspecting a high prevalence of OSA in this group due
to their high BMI and large neck circumference, administered the STOP-
Bang questionnaire and conducted finger pulse oximetry
photoplethysmography-based testing on 56 members of a college
football team. Forty-eight percent of players were determined to be at
high-risk for OSA, and 4 players had AHI of ≥ 5.
Dobrosielski DA et al. Respir Care. 2016 Mar 15.

☐
Smoking significantly increases the risk of sleep apnea. This systematic
review and meta-analysis of longitudinal studies included 216 papers
published to 2013. Other important findings are: (a) risks of lung cancer,
COPD and asthma were increased among adult smokers; (b) smoking,
both active and passive, increased the risk of tuberculosis; and (c) passive
smoke exposure significantly increased the risk of lung cancer in adult
non-smokers, and of asthma, wheezing, lower respiratory tract infections
and diminished lung function in children.
Jayes L et al. Chest. 2016 Apr 18.

☐

Heavy smokers have more severe OSA. A study of 964 patients reported that heavy smokers had higher AHIs compared to mild smokers, and O_2 desaturation time during sleep was significantly longer in former smokers than in never smokers.

Varol Y et al. Sleep Breath. 2015 Dec;19(4):1279-84.

☐

Tooth loss is an independent risk factor for OSA. Researchers reviewed the data from 7,305 adult men and women (aged ≥ 25 years) in the 2005-2008 National Health and Nutrition Examination Survey. Subjects had dental examinations for tooth loss, occlusal contacts and denture use, and were evaluated for OSA using questions based on the AASM criteria. Prevalence of high-risk OSA (≥ 2 signs/symptoms of OSA) increased 2 % for each additional lost tooth. High-risk for OSA was 25% greater in those missing 5-8 teeth, 36% more common in those missing 9-31 teeth, and 61% higher among the edentulous compared to patients with 0-4 lost teeth.

Sanders AE et al. Sleep Breath. 2016 Sep;20(3):1095-102.

☐
Frequent yawning suggests the presence of excessive sleepiness. The frequency of yawning was counted during the day following PSG in 121 snorers. Yawning frequencies in patients with AHI < 5 and AHI > 30 were 43.48 and 75.76, respectively. Frequency of yawning was positively correlated with ESS scores and negatively with mean SaO_2.
Catli T et al. Eur Arch Otorhinolaryngol. 2015 Dec;272(12):3611-5.

☐
There is no significant relationship between AHI and subjective sleepiness or clinical symptoms in middle-aged patients with OSA. Approximately 15.4% of patients studied had moderate-severe OSA (AHI ≥ 15). Impaired vigilance, as assessed by PVT, was present only in those with severe disease (AHI ≥ 30).
Arnardottir ES et al. Eur Respir J. 2015 Nov 5.

☐
Subjective sleep quality, rather than AHI, is the main factor affecting QOL in patients with OSA. Subjects (n = 285) completed questionnaires (PSQI and World Health Organization Quality of Life Short Form) and underwent PSG. In multiple linear regression analysis, the most significant factor associated with QOL was the PSQI total score. The World Health Organization Quality of Life Short Form total score was not related to AHI and its mean score did not differ significantly between patients with OSA vs. simple snorers.
Kang JM et al. Sleep Breath. 2016 Nov 4.

☐
Sleep quality is worse in individuals with upper airway resistance syndrome than in patients with mild OSA. Furthermore, patients with mild OSA had less fatigue and had better sustained attention in the early morning compared to those with upper airway resistance syndrome (UARS). The definition of UARS used in this study was (a) AHI ≤ 5; (b) RDI > 5 or > 30% of TST with flow limitation; and (c) ESS ≥ 10 and/or Modified Fatigue Impact Scale [MFIS] ≥ 38. Investigators performed PVT testing on 34 subjects with UARS, 47 with mild OSA (AHI ≥ 5 and ≤ 15; and ESS ≥ 10 and/or MFIS ≥ 38) and 34 controls (AHI < 5, RDI ≤ 5 and ESS ≤ 9). The

UARS group had worse FOSQ and PSQI scores than the mild OSA group, and scored higher in Beck inventories than controls.
de Godoy LB et al. PLoS One. 2016 May 26;11(5):e0156244.

☐
Cardiovascular and psychiatric comorbidities are more likely to be present in OSA patients with insomnia than in those with EDS. In a prospective cohort study, 6,555 adult OSA patients (AHI ≥ 5) were classified into four phenotypic groups – 20.7% with EDS, 29.8% with insomnia, 23.7% with both EDS and insomnia, and 25.8% with neither EDS nor insomnia. Patients with the insomnia phenotype had a higher prevalence of CV comorbidity than those with the EDS phenotype (56.8% vs. 8.9%), despite the fact that AHI was lower in the insomnia group (27.9 ± 22.5 vs. 35.0 ± 25.5). The insomnia phenotype in OSA patients was associated with psychiatric comorbidity, and the EDS phenotype was associated with higher CPAP use, independent of age, gender or BMI.
Saaresranta T et al. PLoS One. 2016 Oct 4;11(10):e0163439.

☐
The types of major comorbidities in OSA differ between men and women. Analyzing the records from the Truven Health MarketScan Research Databases 2003-2012, a large nationwide U.S. health claims databank of working and retired people with employer-sponsored health insurance, researchers found significant comorbidities in men and women with OSA. Among patients with OSA, type 2 DM and ischemic heart diseases were more prevalent in men, and HTN and depression were more common in women. The gender differences in prevalence of CHF, arrhythmias and stroke were less pronounced.
Mokhlesi B et al. Eur Respir J. 2016 Apr;47(4):1162-9.

☐
Not all patients with positional OSA are alike. Adult patients with positional OSA (n= 1,052) were categorized into 3 groups based on their AHI in a non-supine position: I (non-supine AHI < 5), II (non-supine AHI ≥ 5 and < 15) and III (non-supine AHI ≥ 15). Clinical characteristics for each group were documented. The prevalence of positional OSA was 75.6%, and 39.9% had an AHI < 5 while in a non-supine position. Positional OSA was associated with milder OSA, older age, and lower BMI, but did not influence daytime sleepiness, depressive symptoms, anxiety or HRQOL.

Clinical features did not differ between group III patients and those with non-positional OSA. Supine sleep time was shortest in group III and longest in group I and in those with non-positional OSA.
Lee SA et al. Sleep Breath. 2016 Jul 12.

☐
The two subtypes of positional OSA, namely supine predominant and supine isolated, have different clinical features. Seventy-seven percent of 279 consecutive patients with OSA met criteria for positional OSA, defined as an AHI ≥ 5 with supine AHI twice that of non-supine AHI. Of these, 73.1% had supine predominant OSA, and 26.9% had supine isolated OSA (non-supine AHI < 5). Supine isolated OSA was associated with lower arousal indices, poorer quality of sleep, and more depression and anxiety compared to supine-predominant OSA.
Kim KT et al. Clin Neurophysiol. 2016 Jan;127(1):565-70.

☐
One-third of patients with positional OSA become non-positional during a follow-up PSG. Seventy eight positional OSA patients (i.e., AHI ≥ twice as high in the supine vs. lateral position) underwent a follow-up PSG. Patients were classified as "unchanged" if positional OSA was present in both initial and follow-up PSGs or "changed" if the follow-up PSG demonstrated non-positional OSA. Thirty-five percent of patients converted to non-positional OSA in the second PSG. A higher AI in the lateral position was the only independent predictor of the change to non-positional OSA.
Chou YT et al. J Formos Med Assoc. 2016 Jul 20.

☐
Weight gain continues in obese patients with OSA who are highly adherent to CPAP therapy. Body mass index was measured at baseline and at follow-up visits in 1,023 patients with OSA who were treated with CPAP for an average of 6.6 ± 1.2 years. Mean CPAP usage was 6.0 ± 1.8 hours per day. There was no significant change in BMI in the majority of CPAP-treated patients. Annual weight gain continued in 10% of patients.
Myllylä M et al. J Clin Sleep Med. 2016 Apr 15.

☐
Obstructive sleep apnea can be an early feature of rapid-onset obesity

with hypothalamic dysfunction, hypoventilation and autonomic dysregulation (ROHHAD). This is a retrospective study of 6 children with ROHHAD, a rare disease with a high mortality rate. Polysomnography identified OSA in 66.7% of children, nocturnal hypoventilation in 16.7 %, and both OSA and nocturnal hypoventilation in 16.7%. Polysomnography was repeated in 5 of the 6 children, and all 5 had developed nocturnal hypoventilation and needed NIV at follow-up. Irregular breathing patterns during wakefulness were present in 50% of children.
Reppucci D et al. Orphanet J Rare Dis. 2016 Jul 30;11(1):106.

☐
Chronic rhinosinusitis is common in patients with OSA. In this retrospective cohort study (Taiwan Longitudinal Health Insurance Database 2005), 971 patients with OSA and 4,855 controls were tracked for 5 years. More patients with OSA (6.59%) subsequently developed chronic rhinosinusitis compared with controls (2.00%).
Kao LT et al. Sci Rep. 2016 Feb 10;6:20786.

☐

Middle-aged patients with untreated OSA continue to suffer from worsening AHI and SaO$_2$. This heightened risk was seen even in the absence of weight gain in 82 patients after a mean follow-up of 7.5 years after a diagnostic PSG. Researchers observed significantly longer respiratory event duration and lower SaO$_2$min, but no differences in AHI, baseline SaO2, and 3%ODI, between the baseline and follow-up PSGs. Prolonged respiratory event duration was significantly related to age $\geq$ 60 years and baseline BMI $\geq$ 25, whereas rising AHI was linked to age of 40-60 years and initial OSA severity (mild and moderate). Age of 40-60 years was also significantly associated with lower SaO$_2$min.
Hayashida K et al. Sleep Breath. 2016 May;20(2):711-8.

☐

Risk of all-cause mortality is increased in severe, but not mild-moderate, OSA. Investigators conducted a meta-analysis of 12 prospective cohort studies involving 34,382 subjects, and reported pooled hazard ratios of all-cause mortality of 0.945, 1.178 and 1.601 in those with mild, moderate and severe OSA, respectively.
Pan L et al. Sleep Breath. 2016 Jan 15.

☐

Obstructive sleep apnea increases the risk of postoperative complications. This is a qualitative systematic review conducted by the Society of Anesthesia and Sleep Medicine. Published articles that reported $\geq$ 1 postoperative outcome in adult patients with high risk, or a diagnosis, of OSA who underwent procedures under anesthesia care were collected. These studies included 413,304 patients with OSA and 8,556,279 controls. Pulmonary and combined complications were higher in patients with OSA vs. controls. One study reported an increased in-hospital mortality associated with OSA; in contrast, a decrease in mortality was seen in 3 studies and no change in mortality in 9 studies.
Opperer M et al. Anesth Analg. 2016 May;122(5):1321-34.

☐

A high STOP-Bang score ($\geq$ 3) is associated with an increased risk of perioperative respiratory complications and prolonged length of stay in

patients undergoing urgent surgery. This is a prospective, observational study that assessed if the STOP-Bang questionnaire is able to predict perioperative respiratory complications in 189 adult patients who were having urgent surgery under general anesthesia, of whom 55% had a positive STOP-Bang score (> 3) before anesthesia. The positive STOP-Bang group had more arrhythmias and DM, significantly higher incidence of respiratory complications during surgery and postoperative care period, and prolonged length of hospital stay compared to the negative STOP-Bang group. In a multivariate analysis, the STOP-Bang score was independently correlated with respiratory events.

Chudeau N et al. Anaesth Crit Care Pain Med. 2016 Oct;35(5):347-353.

□
The presence of OSA is not clearly associated with postoperative mortality, cardiopulmonary morbidity, ICU admissions, or length of stay after bariatric surgery. A systematic review of 13 studies, involving 98,935 subjects who had undergone bariatric surgery, was conducted. Thirty-seven percent of the patients had documented OSA. Cardiopulmonary complication rate, which ranged between 0.0% and 25.8%, was not associated with OSA.

de Raaff CA et al. Am J Surg. 2016 Apr;211(4):793-801.

□
Obstructive sleep apnea is associated with significant adverse cognitive effects. Results from 19 studies that utilized objective neuropsychological tests showed significant effects on various cognitive domains, including attention, perception, concept formation, construction, executive functioning, motor control and performance, non-verbal, working and verbal memory, psychomotor speed, speed of processing, and verbal functioning and reasoning.

Stranks EK et al. Arch Clin Neuropsychol. 2016 Jan 6.

□
Obstructive sleep apnea can trigger massive hemoptysis. Researchers reviewed the files of patients who underwent bronchial arterial embolization to treat hemoptysis. Fifty three patients and 58 control subjects were evaluated with PSQI, BQ, STOP and STOP-Bang questionnaires. Hemoptysis requiring re-embolization recurred in 7 patients. High risk of OSA (using BQ) was more common in patients with

hemoptysis than in controls. Percentages of high-risk OSA were 29.7% for those with massive hemoptysis, 12.5% for non-massive hemoptysis and 8.6% for controls. Prevalence of high-risk OSA was 44.4% and 20.5% for patients with idiopathic hemoptysis and with known etiology of hemoptysis, respectively. Lastly, high-risk OSA was also more common in patients who needed re-embolization compared to those who didn't.
Uyar M et al. Sleep Breath. 2016 Dec 19.

☐
Patients with OSA have more than a six-fold higher risk of nonarteritic anterior ischemic optic neuropathy than non-OSA persons. Four prospective cohort studies and 1 case-control study were included in this meta-analysis. Obstructive sleep apnea was a strong independent risk factor of nonarteritic anterior ischemic optic neuropathy, with a pooled odds ratio of 6.18 (95% CI, 2.00-19.11) vs. controls.
Wu Y et al. Curr Eye Res. 2016 Jul;41(7):987-92.

☐
Patients with moderate-severe OSA can develop sensorineural hearing loss. Comprehensive otorhinolaryngological examination, including pure tone auditometry and otoacoustic emission testing, and PSG were performed on 160 patients. Unlike control patients and those with mild OSA who had normal hearing thresholds, patients with moderate-severe OSA had auditory transduction and transmission abnormalities.
Deniz M et al. Am J Otolaryngol. 2016 Jul-Aug;37(4):299-303.

☐
Minimum SaO_2 during PSG is an independent factor affecting hearing in patients with severe OSA. A retrospective review of 41 patients with severe OSA evaluated any association between hypoxia and auditory dysfunction. Hearing was analyzed at a level of ≥ 40 dB. After adjusting for other risk factors of hearing loss, SaO_2min was the only variable that remained significant. Greater severity of O_2 desaturation correlated with worse hearing impairment.
Seo YJ et al. J Clin Sleep Med. 2016 Feb 1.

☐
Abnormal bone metabolism can occur as a consequence of OSA. Bone mineral density and bone turnover markers were measured in 30 men

with OSA (diagnosed by PSG) and 20 healthy men. Bone mineral density measurements and T-scores in the femoral neck were significantly lower, and serum beta-CrossLaps levels were significantly higher, in OSA patients. Both osteocalcin values and neck bone mineral density were significantly related to mean SaO_2 levels.

Terzi R et al. J Bone Miner Metab. 2016 Jul;34(4):475-81.

☐

Patients with OSA, especially those with coexisting DM, have a high risk of developing oral diseases. Among 744 subjects (AHI of 40.9 ± 23.2; BMI of 27.9 ± 5.2; and length of CPAP use of 49.1 ± 30.7 months), 30.4% had halitosis; 27.5% reported gingival bleeding; and 44.6% described having dry mouth since starting CPAP therapy. Compared to non-DM patients, those with DM were significantly older, had higher rate of denture use (28.3 vs. 19.0%), had more frequent dental clinic visits (71.4 vs. 58.7%), and reported more oral symptoms (50.0 vs. 38.2%).

Tsuda H et al. Gerodontology. 2016 Sep;33(3):416-20.

☐

Patients with OSA have higher prevalence of periodontal disease. A case-control study compared the prevalence of periodontitis in 163 individuals (83 patients with OSA and 80 non-OSA controls). Researchers measured clinical periodontal parameters and collected gingival crevicular fluid samples. Patients with OSA had significantly more periodontitis than controls (96.4% vs. 75%, respectively). Prevalence of severe periodontitis as well as gingival crevicular fluid IL-1 beta concentrations and serum high-sensitive CRP levels were also higher in OSA patients compared to controls. Gingival crevicular fluid IL-1 beta and all clinical parameters were significantly correlated. There were no significant inter-group differences in gingival crevicular fluid TNFα and high-sensitive CRP levels.

Gamsiz-Isik H et al. J Periodontol. 2016 Nov 18:1-8.

☐

Obstructive sleep apnea, with or without obesity, increases health resource utilization. Researchers used the 2009-2011 U.S. Nationwide Inpatient Sample of 179,789 adults. Male:female prevalence were: OSA (5.23% vs. 3.88%), obesity (8.95% vs. 17.21%) and both obesity and OSA (6.19% vs. 7.11%). Obstructive sleep apnea and comorbid OSA-obesity were associated with increased health resource utilization and worse inpatient outcomes compared to obesity alone. Patients with OSA, obesity or OSA-obesity had longer hospital length of stays, and increased total hospital charges. Presence of OSA and OSA-obesity increased the need for respiratory therapy.

Becerra MB et al. Respir Med. 2016 Aug;117:230-6.

☐

The risk of MVAs and NMAs among truck drivers is increased by OSA, sleep debt and EDS. Male truck drivers (n = 949) completed a questionnaire about sleep and waking habits, OSA risk factors and EDS. Motor vehicle accidents were reported by 34.8% of participants, and NMAs by 9.2%. Factors that significantly predicted MVAs were OSA, sleep debt and EDS. Sleep debt and OSA increased the risk of NMAs. Talking naps or rest breaks prevented both MVAs and NMAs.

Garbarino S et al. PLoS One. 2016 Nov 30;11(11):e0166262.

☐

Seven percent of road traffic injuries from MVAs among male drivers are related to OSA. The proportion of road traffic injuries attributable to OSA can be assessed using the population attributable fraction (PAF), which combines the prevalence of OSA and OSA-dependent MVA odds ratio. Using this formula, 7% of road traffic injuries from MVAs among male drivers were estimated to be due to OSA.

Garbarino S et al. Chron Respir Dis. 2015 Nov;12(4):320-8.

☐

The number of serious preventable truck crashes increases fivefold in patients who are non-adherent to OSA therapy. Analyzing data from an employer-mandated program that screens, diagnoses and monitors treatment adherence of OSA in the U.S. trucking industry, investigators conducted a retrospective cohort of 1,614 patients with OSA, 403 non-OSA controls and 2,016 drivers who were unlikely to have OSA. Patients with OSA were treated with APAP and adherence to therapy was classified as full, partial or none. The rate of preventable crashes per 100,000 miles in the fully adherent group was statistically similar to controls.

Burks SV et al. Sleep. 2016 May 1;39(5):967-75.

☐

Accidents due to falling asleep at the wheel are related to subjective reports of feeling drowsy during regular driving and working. The authors investigated the risk factors for automobile accidents caused by falling asleep while driving in patients with OSA. Multivariate analysis of 2,387 subjects with OSA and 394 simple snorers revealed that ESS scores and self-reported frequency of feeling drowsy during regular driving and working were important. Rates of drowsy driving and of accidents due to falling asleep were significantly higher in subjects with very severe OSA (AHI ≥ 60) compared to snorers and subjects with less severe OSA.
Arita A et al. Sleep Breath. 2015 Dec;19(4):1229-34.

☐

Workers with OSA are at risk for occupational accidents. Seven studies were included in this meta-analysis on the relationship between OSA and work-related accidents. The odds of work accident were nearly double in workers with OSA compared to non-OSA controls.
Garbarino S et al. Sleep. 2016 Jun 1;39(6):1211-8.

☐

Patients with OSA are at risk for occupational injury. Canadian researchers reported the frequency and types of occupational injuries in the 5 years prior to PSG among 1,236 patients who had been referred to the sleep laboratory for evaluation of suspected OSA. Compared to controls, patients with OSA were twice more likely to have had at least one occupational injury and almost three times the chance of having an injury related to reduced vigilance. However, these associations were reduced after controlling for confounders.
Hirsch Allen AJ et al. Thorax. 2016 Mar 15.

☐
Objective daytime sleepiness in OSA patients increases the likelihood of developing HTN. Polysomnography followed by MSLT was performed on 1,338 patients with OSA and 484 primary snorers. Compared with the primary snorer group that had an MSLT > 8 minutes, and after controlling for confounders, OSA plus MSLT of 5-8 minutes and MSLT < 5 minutes increased the odds of HTN by 95% and 111%, respectively.
Ren R et al. Hypertension. 2016 Nov;68(5):1264-1270.

☐
Mean apnea-hypopnea duration, but not AHI, heightens the likelihood of moderate-severe HTN in patients with OSA. In a retrospective study, possible relationships between various PSG parameters and severity of HTN were assessed in 596 patients with HTN and OSA (AHI ≥ 5 based on PSG). Longer mean apnea-hypopnea duration, but not AHI, ODI, or lowest SaO_2, was significantly related to more severe HTN. In addition, mean apnea-hypopnea duration was independently associated with moderate-severe HTN.
Wu H et al. Medicine (Baltimore). 2016 Nov;95(48):e5493.

☐
Isolated REM sleep OSA can give rise to HTN. As part of the Men Androgens Inflammation Lifestyle Environment and Stress (MAILES) Study, 837 community-dwelling men without a prior diagnosis of OSA (AHI < 10) underwent full in-home PSG. Severe REM OSA [AHI ≥ 30] had independent adjusted associations with prevalent HTN at follow-up (related to their OSA status) and recent-onset HTN at follow-up (in men without HTN at baseline). No association was observed between HTN and non-REM AHI.
Appleton SL et al. Chest. 2016 Mar 18. pii: S0012-3692(16)41674-0.

☐
Short-term CPAP therapy reduces systolic and diastolic BP in OSA patients with controlled HTN. Thirty six patients with HTN controlled using oral antihypertensive medications and recently diagnosed OSA were enrolled in a prospective cohort study. Systolic and diastolic BP were recorded using 24-hour ambulatory BP measurements at baseline

and after 5 days of CPAP use. Significant reductions in mean 24-hour systolic BP and diastolic BP were seen.

de Morais Lima JH et al. Postgrad Med J. 2016 Mar;92(1085):134-6.

☐

Long-term PAP therapy lowers BP in OSA patients with and without coexisting HTN. Blood pressure was measured at baseline and after 2 years of PAP treatment in 1,168 patients with newly diagnosed OSA. Significant reductions in systolic and diastolic BP were seen at follow-up in patients with and without HTN. The magnitude of change in systolic and diastolic BP was correlated with hours of PAP use.

Bouloukaki I et al. J Hum Hypertens. 2016 Jul 28.

☐

Positive airway pressure therapy reduces nighttime BP surges in patients with OSA and OHS. Nocturnal beat-to-beat BP surges were evaluated in 17 OHS patients with OSA who each underwent PSG and finger plethysmography. The number of BP surges per hour decreased during PAP titration and 6 weeks of PAP treatment. The latter also lowered mean nocturnal BP but not daytime BP. Adherence to therapy correlated positively to improved BP control.

Carter JR et al. Am J Physiol Regul Integr Comp Physiol. 2016 Apr 1;310(7):R602-11.

☐

Treating OSA with CPAP in patients with BP-controlled HTN converts "non-dippers" to "dippers". Seventeen patients with severe OSA (AHI > 30) underwent PSG before and after ≈ 8 weeks of CPAP treatment, and their motor activity and circadian rhythms of BP, HR, plasma norepinephrine and plasma melatonin were measured. Continuous positive airway pressure therapy increased the number of BP "dippers", lowered 24-hour plasma norepinephrine values, and improved AHI, ODI, arousal index, N3 sleep and REM sleep, but did not significantly change the level and rhythm of BP and HR, or the disturbed circadian pattern of melatonin.

Lemmer B et al. Blood Press Monit. 2016 Jun;21(3):136-43.

☐

Therapy with CPAP favorably reduces BP in OSA patients with resistant

HTN. In a meta-analysis of 5 RCTs published before March 20, 2015, CPAP therapy was associated with reductions in nocturnal diastolic BP and in 24-hr ambulatory systolic and diastolic BP.

Liu L et al. J Clin Hypertens (Greenwich). 2016 Feb;18(2):153-8.

☐

Fixed-pressure CPAP is more effective than APAP in reducing 24-hr diastolic BP, but not office systolic BP, in patients with OSA. A double-blind RCT was conducted to study the impact of 4 months of CPAP vs. APAP therapy on BP control in 322 patients. Median device use was 5.1 hours per night. Reduction in systolic BP was not significantly different between the CPAP and APAP groups (2.2 vs. 0.4 mmHg), but diastolic BP decreased by 1.7 mmHg in the CPAP group and by 0.5 mmHg in the APAP group.

Pépin JL et al. Thorax. 2016 Aug;71(8):726-33.

☐

Blood pressure increases when CPAP therapy for OSA is discontinued. The rise in BP was positively correlated with worse OSA severity. Data from 3 RCTs, of 149 CPAP-complaint patients with OSA who were randomized to either continue or discontinue therapy for 2 weeks, were analyzed. Withdrawal of CPAP led to an increase in AHI (2.8 at baseline vs. 33.2 at follow-up) and significantly higher systolic and diastolic BPs. In multivariate analysis, AHI was independently associated with the change in systolic BP.

Schwarz EI et al. Chest. 2016 Dec;150(6):1202-1210.

☐

Oxygen desaturation index independently predicts an elevated risk of CV disease. The Taiwan Bus Driver Cohort Study, which consisted of 1,014 professional drivers, was linked to the National Health Insurance Research Dataset of 192 cases of CV disease. The researchers wanted to determine if overnight pulse oximetry and 8-year risk of CV disease are related. After adjusting for CV risk factors, both 4%ODI ($\geq$ 6.5) and 3%ODI ($\geq$ 10) increased 8-year CV risk.

Wu WT et al. Int J Cardiol. 2016 Dec 15;225:206-212.

☐

Continuous positive airway pressure therapy does not decrease the risk of CV events. Eighteen RCTs (4,146 patients) were included in this meta-analysis. Compared to controls, CPAP significantly lowered 24-hour systolic and diastolic BP as well as ESS, but had no impact on CV events, death, or stroke.

Guo J et al. Sleep Breath. 2016 Feb 12.

☐

Moderate-severe OSA can independently lead to subclinical coronary atherosclerosis in middle-aged women. Subclinical atherosclerosis was assessed by tomographic coronary calcium score in 214 middle-aged perimenopausal or postmenopausal women without known CV disease. Obstructive sleep apnea (AHI ≥ 5) was diagnosed in 38% of the subjects using portable sleep studies. Prevalence of coronary artery calcium was higher in subjects with moderate-severe OSA (AHI ≥ 15) than in those with no or mild OSA.

Medeiros AK et al. Sleep Breath. 2016 Jul 6.

☐

Severe OSA causes overnight myocardial injury in patients with refractory angina. Markers of myocardial injury (including blood high-sensitivity cardiac troponin T [hs-cTnT]) were obtained at 14:00, 22:00 and 7:00 in 80 patients with refractory angina. Subjects also underwent overnight PSG and imaging stress tests by single-photon emission computed tomography (SPECT) and/or cardiac MRI. Seventy-five percent of the patients had OSA (AHI > 15). Morning peak of hs-cTnT was two times higher in patients with AHI ≥ 51 compared to the remaining population.

Geovanini GR et al. Heart. 2016 Apr 5.

☐

There is a high prevalence of SDB in patients with acute coronary syndrome. A meta-analysis of 32 studies was conducted to review the prevalence of SDB in 3,360 patients with acute coronary syndrome. The pooled prevalence was 69% for all SDB (AHI > 5), 43% for moderate-severe SDB (AHI > 15), and 25% for severe SDB (AHI > 30). The pooled prevalence was similar for Western and Asian populations.

Huang Z et al. Sleep Breath. 2016 Aug 22.

☐
Moderate-severe OSA confers a worse survival among patients with acute coronary syndrome. In a prospective longitudinal cohort study, cardiorespiratory sleep study and/or PSG were performed in 73 patients admitted for an acute coronary syndrome. Prevalence of OSA was 63% in this population (mild OSA in 30% and moderate-severe OSA in 70%). After a median follow-up period of 75 months, those with moderate-severe OSA had a lower event-free survival rate and a higher incidence in the composite end point of death for any cause, MI and need for myocardial revascularization. Unfortunately, compliance to CPAP therapy had no impact on the composite end point.
Leão S et al. Am J Cardiol. 2016 Apr 1;117(7):1084-7.

☐
Nocturnal hypoxemia related to OSA worsens the prognosis after an MI. Researchers conducted a prospective study involving 112 subjects with no prior history of sleep apnea, who underwent PSG after having had an MI. Those with CSA or who were using CPAP were excluded. Prevalence of OSA (AHI ≥ 15) was 41%. Subjects were followed for 48 months. Rates of major adverse cardiac events were significantly higher in the OSA group compared to the non-OSA group, and nocturnal SaO_2min ≤ 85% was an independent risk factor for major adverse cardiac events.
Xie J, Sert Kuniyoshi FH et al. J Am Heart Assoc. 2016 Jul 27;5(8).

☐
Sleep disordered breathing increases the incidence of major adverse cardio-cerebrovascular events in patients with acute coronary syndrome following primary percutaneous coronary intervention. Sleep disordered breathing (AHI ≥ 5 by overnight cardiorespiratory monitoring) was present in 52.3% of 241 patients with acute coronary syndrome who successfully underwent primary percutaneous coronary intervention. Over a median follow-up period of 5.6 years, the cumulative incidence of major adverse cardio-cerebrovascular events, including a composite of all-cause death, recurrence of acute coronary syndrome, nonfatal stroke and hospital admission for HF, was significantly higher in SDB patients than in the non-SDB group. Multivariable analysis showed that SDB was a significant predictor of major adverse cardio-cerebrovascular events.
Mazaki T et al. J Am Heart Assoc. 2016 Jun 15;5(6).

☐

There is a high prevalence of SDB in patients with stable chronic HF. In this prospective multicenter registry (SchlaHF; Sleep-Disordered Breathing in Heart Failure), which involved 6,876 symptomatic patients with chronic, but stable, HF (NYHA class ≥ II; LVEF ≤ 45%), the prevalence of moderate-severe SDB (AHI ≥ 15) was 46%. Risk factors for SDB were male gender, weight (BMI), increasing age, lower LVEF, and AF.
Arzt M et al. JACC Heart Fail. 2015 Dec 7.

☐

Risk of incident or decompensated HF is heightened in older men who have an elevated CAI or CSR, but not in those with an elevated OAHI. In a prospective multicenter observational study of community-dwelling older men (Osteoporotic Fractures in Men Study), 2,865 participants underwent PSG and were followed for a mean of 7.3 years for the development of incident or decompensated HF. Unlike OAHI, a CAI ≥ 5 and the presence of CSR were significant predictors of incident HF. If patients with baseline HF were excluded, incident risk of HF remained significantly elevated in patients with CSR.
Javaheri S et al. Am J Respir Crit Care Med. 2016 Mar 1;193(5):561-8.

☐

Nocturnal hypoxia is an independent predictor of all-cause mortality in patients with CHF and OSA. In this prospective cohort study, 963 HF patients with reduced LVEF (NYHA class ≥ II) underwent polygraphy. During follow-up for a median of 7.35 years, 49.8% of the patients died. Mortality rate was 8.1 and 12.2% in those with no/mild and moderate-severe OSA, respectively. Time with SaO_2 < 90%, but not AHI, was significantly associated with time to death from any cause even after adjustment for confounding factors. The risk of death increased by 16.1% per hour of time with SaO_2 < 90%.
Oldenburg O et al. Eur Heart J. 2016 Jun 1;37(21):1695-703.

☐

Obstructive sleep apnea worsens long-term cardiac function and outcomes in HF patients with preserved ejection fraction. This negative impact was seen even in patients whose OSA was appropriately treated. Levels of BNP were obtained in 58 patients with HF (LVEF ≥ 50%) at baseline, and at 1, 6, 12 and 36 months. Sixty-seven percent of subjects had OSA (diagnosed with PSG) and were treated with CPAP. Baseline E/E' on echocardiography tended to be higher, but median BNP levels were similar, in the OSA vs. non-OSA groups. Levels of BNP decreased over time in both groups, but the change was less pronounced in patients with OSA, who had higher BNP levels at 6, 12 and 36 months.

Arikawa T et al. Heart Lung Circ. 2016 May;25(5):435-41.

☐

Obstructive sleep apnea, by itself, decreases LV systolic and RV function. Investigators of the Wisconsin Sleep Cohort Study performed transthoracic echocardiography on 601 persons with OSA at 18.0 ± 3.7 years after PSG. After adjustment for age, gender and BMI, baseline AHI was related significantly and progressively with future reduced LVEF and RV function (tricuspid annular plane systolic excursion (TAPSE) ≤ 15 mm). Indices of O_2 desaturation were independently associated with LV mass, LV wall thickness and RV area.

Korcarz CE et al. Sleep. 2016 Apr 12.

☐

The proportion of recording time containing 4% desaturation events (4%POD), a measure of nocturnal hypoxemic burden, is an independent predictor of mortality in HF patients with CSA. The authors of the study prospectively performed cardiorespiratory polygraphy on 112 HF patients with systolic or diastolic dysfunction. Central sleep apnea was diagnosed if AHI ≥ 5 events; and > 75% of events were central. Twenty-nine percent of the subjects died during a follow-up period of 37 ± 25 months. The 4%POD was the best independent predictor of mortality. A higher 4%POD, but not AHI or proportion of sleep time with SaO_2 < 90%, was seen in non-survivors compared to survivors.

Watanabe E et al. J Card Fail. 2016 Sep 9.

☐

Obstructive sleep apnea is a risk factor for AF independent of other risk factors. Of 6,841 subjects, 455 developed AF during a median follow-up of 11.9 years. Independent predictors of incident AF included AHI > 5 and time with SaO_2 < 90%.

Cadby G et al. Chest. 2015 Oct 1;148(4):945-52.

☐
Central sleep apnea and CSR predict a heightened risk of new-onset AF in older men. Which indices of SDB can predict incident AF? To answer this question, researchers conducted sleep studies on 843 ambulatory older men without AF. Subjects were followed for 6.5 ± 0.7 years to identify incident AF. Both CSA and CSA/CSR, but not obstructive apnea or hypoxemia, predicted incident AF. Atrial fibrillation was related to CSA, CSA/CSR and AHI among subjects aged ≥ 76 years.
May AM et al. Am J Respir Crit Care Med. 2016 Apr 1;193(7):783-91.

☐
Continuous positive airway pressure therapy for OSA decreases risk of AF. This meta-analysis consisted of 8 studies involving 698 CPAP users and 549 non-CPAP users. Patients who were treated with CPAP had a 42% lower risk of AF. Benefits of CPAP therapy were more pronounced in male, younger and obese patients.
Qureshi WT et al. Am J Cardiol. 2015 Dec 1;116(11):1767-73.

☐
Continuous positive airway pressure therapy does not affect ECG markers of AF and sudden cardiac death risk in patients with minimally symptomatic OSA. The MOSAIC (Multicentre Obstructive Sleep Apnoea Interventional Cardiovascular) trial randomized 303 patients with minimally symptomatic OSA (mean baseline ODI of 13.1 ± 12.3) to CPAP or standard care for 6 months. Full 12-lead ECG data were available in 250 patients. Continuous positive airway pressure had no impact on risk markers for AF and sudden cardiac death.
Schlatzer C et al. BMJ Open. 2016 Mar 16;6(3):e010150.

☐
Aortic stiffness, which is associated with higher risk of CV morbidity and deaths, increases proportionately to AHI severity in OSA patients. Aortic pulse wave velocity, augmentation index and aortic distensibility were calculated in 90 patients with OSA (diagnosed with PSG). Subjects were classified as having low AHI or high AHI. Those with high AHI had lower aortic distensibility values and higher pulse wave velocity values. Apnea hypopnea index was independently associated with pulse wave velocity and aortic distensibility in multivariate linear regression analysis.
Çörtük M et al. Clin Respir J. 2016 Jul;10(4):455-61.

☐
Peripheral arterial occlusive disease is significantly associated with OSA.
A nationwide population-based case-control study consisted of 11,817
patients with peripheral arterial occlusive disease and 35,451 controls.
The association between OSA and peripheral arterial occlusive disease
was noted in both univariate and multivariate logistic regression
analyses, which adjusted for CAD or MI, CKD, hyperuricemia and obesity.
This association was lessened when further adjusted for HTN, DM and
hyperlipidemia.
Chen JC et al. Clin Otolaryngol. 2015 Oct;40(5):437-42.

☐
**Minimum, but not mean, nocturnal SaO$_2$ independently predicts future
carotid atherosclerosis.** Data from the Wisconsin Sleep Cohort Study on
689 subjects who underwent a baseline PSG followed by carotid
ultrasonography 7.8 years (mean) later demonstrated that SaO$_2$min
predicted future carotid artery plaque score even after adjustment for
traditional CV risk factors.
Gunnarsson SI et al. J Sleep Res. 2015 Dec;24(6):680-6.

☐
**Continuous positive airway pressure therapy decreases arterial stiffness
in patients with HTN and OSA.** Arterial stiffness is a known predictor of
all-cause and CV mortality in patients with HTN. The investigators
conducted a meta-analysis of 3 articles with 186 patients, and concluded
that arterial stiffness was significantly decreased by CPAP.
Lin X et al. Eur Arch Otorhinolaryngol. 2016 Feb 9.

☐
**Brain damage can occur with OSA as can partial recovery of
nonpermanent structural damage with long-term CPAP treatment.**
Neuroimaging evidence of widespread neocortical and cerebellar atrophy
in untreated patients, and increases in brain volume following therapy in
21 patients with OSA may reflect compensatory neurogenesis.
Kim H et al. Hum Brain Mapp. 2015 Oct 27.

☐
Risk of incident stroke is increased in older men with severe nocturnal

hypoxemia. Metrics of OSA, including AHI, OAHI, CAI and nocturnal hypoxemia, were measured during PSG in 2,872 community-dwelling older men (mean age of 76 years) who were enrolled in the MrOS Sleep Study. Incident stroke occurred in 5.4% of the patients over an average follow-up period of 7.3 years. Compared to patients with normal nighttime O_2 levels, those with severe nocturnal hypoxemia ($\geq$ 10% of the night with SaO_2 < 90%) had a 1.8-fold increased risk of incident stroke. Incident stroke was not associated with AHI, OAHI or CAI.
Stone KL et al. Sleep. 2016 Mar 1;39(3):531-40.

☐
Wake-up stroke in men is linked to severity of OSA and degree of O_2 desaturation. About one in four ischemic strokes are considered wake-up strokes (WUS). Subjects in the Sleep Apnea in Transient Ischemic Attack and Stroke (SLEEP TIGHT) Study underwent PSG and ambulatory BP monitoring. Thirty percent of 164 subjects had WUS. Higher rates of severe OSA (AHI > 30) and more 3% O_2 desaturation events were noted in men, but in not women, with WUS.
Koo BB et al. Cerebrovasc Dis. 2016 Jan 27;41(5-6):233-241.

☐
Obstructive sleep apnea is more common in patients with TIA than in those without vascular disease. Five hundred and fifty five patients suspected of having a TIA were screened for OSA using 3 factors, namely the presence of snoring, ESS > 10 and BMI $\geq$ 30. Polysomnography was performed in 77 patients who had $\geq$ 2 positive factors. Patients with TIA had nearly twice the prevalence of OSA (AHI $\geq$ 5) than patients without vascular disease (80% vs. 47%).
Schipper MH et al. J Stroke Cerebrovasc Dis. 2016 Mar 7.

☐
Obstructive sleep apnea accelerates the decline of kidney function.
During a 10-year period, 6,866 subjects with OSA and controls matched
for age, sex, DM and HTN were followed for the development of new
CKD. Median duration to development of CKD was 2.5 months earlier in
the OSA group than in controls.
Lin YS et al. Sleep Breath. 2016 Jul 5.

☐
Risk of incident CKD is heightened by sleep apnea. This retrospective
cohort study involved 8,687 adult patients with newly diagnosed sleep
apnea and 34,747 matched subjects without sleep apnea. During a mean
follow-up period of 3.9 years, 157 and 298 new CKD events (incidence
rates of 4.5 and 2.2 per 1000 person-years) were recorded in patients
with and without sleep apnea, respectively. Increased risk due to sleep
apnea was similar to that from HTN but was less than from DM.
Chu H et al. Respirology. 2016 Jan 22.

☐
Men with OSA have a higher likelihood of having urological disorders. A
population-based cross-sectional study, which used the Taiwan
Longitudinal Health Insurance Database 2005, revealed that men with
OSA had significantly more prostate diseases (hypertrophy, chronic
prostatitis and cancer), nocturia, urinary diseases (incontinence and
calculi) and erectile dysfunction compared to men without OSA.
Chung SD et al. Sleep Breath 2016 Apr 7.

☐
**Sleep disordered breathing is frequently present in patients
complaining of nocturia.** Sleep disordered breathing (3% ODI > 5) was
present in 70.6% of 34 patients who visited a urology clinic complaining
of nocturia. Therapy with CPAP reduced the frequency of nighttime
urination in patients who were previously resistant to conventional
medical therapy.
Yamamoto U et al. Intern Med. 2016;55(8):901-5.

☐
Obstructive sleep apnea and circadian changes in extracellular fluid contribute to the development of nocturnal polyuria. Morning and night body fluid composition (using bioelectric impedance analysis) and voiding frequency and volume (24-h frequency-volume chart) were recorded in 22 patients with OSA after CPAP therapy. Multivariate linear regression analysis demonstrated an independent relationship between nocturnal polyuria and (a) AHI and (b) circadian change in extracellular fluid adjusted to lean body mass. Significant improvements in nocturia related to CPAP use were observed only in patients with nocturnal polyuria.
Niimi A et al. J Urol. 2016 Apr 19.

☐
The possibility of comorbid OSA should be considered when evaluating men presenting with complaints of nocturia. Nocturia (i.e., ≥ 2 voids per main sleep period) was assessed in 708 men without prostate or bladder cancer and/or surgery, and no prior OSA diagnosis. Those with nocturia had high levels of OSA (32.2%), increased WASO, less N2 and REM sleep, poor sleep quality and more EDS. Nocturia was positively associated with OSA, EDS and worse sleep quality in multiple-adjusted models.
Martin SA et al. Urology. 2016 Jun 24.

☐
Erectile dysfunction is more common in OSA than non-OSA patients, and is improved by CPAP therapy. Patients with OSA also had lower sex hormone levels than controls. Investigators obtained PSG data, International Index of Erectile Dysfunction-5 (IIEF) scores, and blood samples from 153 OSA patients and 60 healthy controls. Prevalence of erectile dysfunction was 47.1% in OSA patients and 13.3% in controls. Patients with OSA and erectile dysfunction had lower serum levels of follicle stimulating hormone (FSH) and testosterone than OSA patients without erectile dysfunction. The IIEF-5 score, sex hormone levels and PSG were repeated in 32 patients with severe OSA and erectile dysfunction following 1 month of CPAP treatment. Therapy with CPAP increased serum levels of FSH, luteinizing hormone and testosterone, and improved the symptoms of erectile dysfunction (IIEF score).
Li Z et al. Respir Med. 2016 Oct;119:130-134.

☐
Nasal CPAP treatment of OSA improves sexual function among male patients and their female partners. Sexual functioning was evaluated prospectively in 21 male patients with moderate-severe OSA and erectile dysfunction and their female partners before and after 12 weeks of CPAP therapy. Treatment was associated with significantly higher scores of the International Index of Erectile Function (IIEF) among men and the Female Sexual Function Index in women.
Acar M et al. Eur Arch Otorhinolaryngol. 2016 Jan;273(1):133-7.

☐
Obstructive sleep apnea heightens the possibility of developing metabolic syndrome independent of obesity. This conclusion was reached using a meta-analysis of 13 studies, including 3 case-control studies (n = 857) and 10 cross-sectional studies (n = 7,077). Increased metabolic risk was significantly associated with OSA, ODI and percentage of sleep time with SaO_2 < 90%.
Qian Y et al. Arch Med Sci. 2016 Oct 1;12(5):1077-1087.

☐
Nocturnal hypoxemia leads to hyperglycemia in patients with OSA and type 2 DM. The relationship between SaO_2 and interstitial glucose level (IGL) was studied in 130 patients who each underwent PSG and oral glucose tolerance tests. Several variables, including AHI, mean SaO_2, SaO_2min and microarousal index were associated with higher IGL.
Hui P et al. Am J Med Sci. 2016 Feb;351(2):160-8.

☐
Severe OSA increases the likelihood of developing DM independent of obesity. Middle-aged and older non-diabetic subjects enrolled in the Atherosclerosis Risk in Communities Study and the Sleep Heart Health Study (n = 1,453) underwent PSG testing. There were 285 cases of incident DM cases identified by telephone calls during a median follow-up of 13 years. Patients with severe OSA (AHI ≥ 30) had a greater risk of incident DM compared to normal controls (AHI < 5) even after accounting for differences in BMI and waist circumference.
Nagayoshi M et al. Sleep Med. 2016 Sep;25:156-161.

☐

Continuous positive airway pressure therapy reduces insulin resistance in non-diabetic and pre-diabetic patients with OSA. A meta-analysis of 23 studies (19 prospective studies and 4 RCTs), which included 965 patients with OSA, confirmed that CPAP therapy significantly reduced insulin resistance (homeostasis model assessment of insulin resistance [HOMA-IR]) vs. controls. The 2 groups had similar changes in fasting blood glucose and fasting insulin compared to baseline levels. For RCT studies, CPAP therapy significantly reduced fasting insulin, but not HOMA-IR or fasting blood glucose.
Chen L et al. Eur J Intern Med. 2016 Nov 30.

☐

Using CPAP for 8 hours per night over a course of 1 week improves glycemic control in patients with OSA. Twelve subjects with DM type 2 and OSA were evaluated before and after 1 week of an entire 8-hour-night CPAP therapy. Levels of glucose, insulin and counter-regulatory hormones were measured every 15 to 30 minutes for 24 hours under controlled conditions. Using CPAP reduced 24-hour mean glucose, morning fasting glucose levels, dawn phenomenon and norepinephrine levels, but did not change 24-hour profiles of growth hormone and cortisol.
Mokhlesi B et al. Diabetes Obes Metab. 2016 Nov 17.

☐

Continuous positive airway pressure treatment improves insulin resistance and glycemic control in patients with OSA and suboptimally controlled type 2 DM. In this 6-month RCT, 50 subjects with OSA and type 2 DM, in whom glycated hemoglobin (HbA1c) levels were ≥ 6.5% on 2 occasions, were randomized to CPAP or no CPAP. Insulin resistance and sensitivity, HbA1c, and serum levels of IL-1β, IL-6 and adiponectin improved after 6 months in the CPAP group.
Martínez-Cerón E et al. Am J Respir Crit Care Med. 2016 Feb 24.

☐

In contrast to its beneficial effect on glycemic control in poorly controlled type 2 DM, CPAP therapy for OSA does not improve glucose levels in those with well-controlled type 2 DM. Four hundred and sixteen diabetic patients (HbA1c level of 6.5-8.5%) and ODI ≥ 15 were assigned to receive PAP or no PAP therapy. Change in HbA1c did not differ between the study groups.

Shaw JE et al. Am J Respir Crit Care Med. 2016 Aug 15;194(4):486-92.

☐
Twenty-four hour cortisol levels are significantly higher in patients with OSA compared to controls, and are lowered by CPAP therapy. Investigators studied 35 subjects with OSA and 37 controls in the sleep laboratory for 4 nights. Blood was sampled every hour for 24 hours on the 4th day and night at baseline and at 2 months after CPAP or sham-CPAP treatment. In nonobese men and slightly obese women, OSA is associated with increased cortisol levels suggesting an activation of the hypothalamic-pituitary-adrenal (HPA) axis.

Kritikou I et al. Eur Respir J. 2016 Feb;47(2):531-40.

☐
Hypothyroidism influences the severity of OSA. This meta-analysis included 12 studies and 5 case reports that involved 192 hypothyroid patients with OSA and 1,423 euthyroid patients with OSA. At the time of OSA diagnosis, AHI, time of sleep with SaO_2 < 90% and ESS were significantly higher in the hypothyroid vs. euthyroid group, but there were no significant inter-group differences in RDI, SE or arousal index.

Zhang M et al. Curr Med Res Opin. 2016 Jun;32(6):1059-64.

☐
Sleep disordered breathing increases the risk of incident cancer. This meta-analysis of 5 studies involved 34,848 patients with SDB/OSA and 77,380 patients without SDB. Patients with SDB/OSA had a higher likelihood of having incident cancer when adjusted for traditional cancer risk factors. The percentage of patients with and without SDB who developed incident cancers was 1.6% and 0.37%, respectively.

Palamaner Subash Shantha G et al. Sleep Med. 2015 Oct;16(10):1289-94.

☐
Obstructive sleep apnea increases the risk of certain cancers (pancreatic, kidney and melanoma) but does not increase the likelihood of metastatic cancer or cancer-related deaths. A large national health insurance database of an estimated 5.6 million individuals was analyzed for the incidence of 12 major cancer types in patients with OSA. Another

cohort of patients with cancer was used to assess the risk of metastases or mortality from cancer in OSA patients. The incidence of all cancer diagnoses combined was similar in OSA and non-OSA patients. Adjusted risk of three cancers (pancreatic, kidney and melanoma) was significantly higher, and the risk of colorectal, breast and prostate cancers were lower in patients with OSA. Obstructive sleep apnea was not associated with an increased risk for metastasis or death in patients with cancer.
Gozal D et al. Sleep. 2016 Aug 1;39(8):1493-500.

☐
Risk for comorbid OSA is present in 29% of adults meeting epidemiological criteria for COPD. Researchers in Taiwan carried out a random cross-sectional national telephone survey and compared the data from COPD cases with and without risk of OSA. The overall prevalence of COPD in this national sample was 6.1%. The group at risk for OSA had significantly higher BMI and COPD Assessment Test scores, and were more likely to have HTN or CV disease, DM and performance impairment than those who were not at risk for OSA.
Hang LW et al. Int J Chron Obstruct Pulmon Dis. 2016 Mar 30;11:665-73.

☐
Overlap syndrome is likely even in COPD patients who have *no* symptoms of OSA. Overlap syndrome is characterized by the co-occurrence of OSA and COPD. This article reported the prevalence of this syndrome in 45 patients with mild hypoxemic COPD and no OSA symptoms. Polygraphy and laboratory testing were performed. Fifty-eight percent of patients had an RDI of ≥ 15. A significant correlation was found between RDI and BMI, and a BMI > 27 had a sensitivity and specificity of 73% and 68%, respectively, for identifying overlap syndrome.
Basoglu OK et al. Clin Respir J. 2016 May 5.

☐
Worse emphysema and gas trapping are linked to decreased AHI among OSA patients who smoke. Fifty one participants (BMI 32 ± 9) of the Genetic Epidemiology of COPD (COPDGene) project underwent full-night PSG. The prevalence of OSA was 57%. Compared to subjects without OSA, those with OSA were younger and had higher BMI. Factors linked to AHI included computed tomography (CT)-derived percent emphysema and

CT-derived percent gas trapping, suggesting that lung inflation may be an important determinant of UA stability in patients with OSA.

Krachman SL et al. Ann Am Thorac Soc. 2016 Jul;13(7):1129-35.

☐

Patients with overlap syndrome have heightened cardiac sympathetic activity compared to patients with either OSA or COPD alone. Heart rate variability was evaluated in 14, 24 and 16 patients with overlap syndrome, OSA and COPD, respectively. Significantly lower high-frequency (0.4-0.15 Hz) power, greater low-frequency (0.15-0.05 Hz) power, and higher LF/HF ratio were observed in the overlap group compared with either COPD and OSA groups – findings that are consistent with higher sympathetic modulation of HR variability.

Taranto-Montemurro L et al. COPD. 2016 Jul 6:1-6.

☐

Early recognition and effective treatment of OSA in patients hospitalized for COPD exacerbation reduce hospital readmissions. Mean clinical events (hospital admissions and emergency room visits) in 24 patients decreased following intervention compared to the same time period prior to therapy if they were compliant to PAP therapy at 6 months (-2.1 ± 0.3) and 12 months (-2.7 ± 0.5) but not if they were non-complaint (-0.8 ± 0.5 and -0.8 ± 0.6, respectively).

Konikkara J et al. Hosp Pract. 2016;44(1):41-7.

☐

Increasing severity of SDB diminishes the incremental impact of worsening lung function on all-cause mortality. Investigators determined the association between mortality, lung function and severity of SDB in 6,173 participants of the Sleep Heart Health Study. All-cause mortality rate was 26.9 and 18.2 per 1,000 person-years in those with SDB (AHI ≥ 5) and without SDB, respectively. Worse lung function was associated with a higher risk for all-cause mortality. For every 200-ml decrease in FEV_1, all-cause mortality increased by 11.0% in those without SDB but by only 6.0% in the SDB group.

Putcha N et al. Am J Respir Crit Care Med. 2016 Oct 15;194(8):1007-1014.

☐

Risk of OSA is increased in current asthma patients and in women with

chronic airflow limitation. Adults (n = 3506) living in Norway completed a questionnaire on medical, sleep and respiratory history and underwent spirometry testing. Prevalence of OSA (defined by positive answers to questions) was higher among middle-aged subjects (6.2%) vs. older adults (3.6%). Obstructive sleep apnea was more prevalent in those who reported respiratory symptoms. Significant associations with OSA included current asthma, lowest quartile of post-bronchodilator FVC, and post-bronchodilator $FEV_1/FVC < 0.7$ [the latter only in women].
Jonassen TM et al. Clin Respir J. 2016 Mar 7.

☐
Therapy with CPAP reduces asthma symptoms in OSA patients with coexisting asthma. A survey questionnaire, which included a Finnish version of the Asthma Control Test (ACT) and a visual analogue scale, was sent to 2,577 patients with OSA who were being treated with CPAP. Prevalence of asthma among the 1,586 respondents was 13%. Initiation of CPAP while on asthma medications increased ACT scores, decreased self-reported asthma severity, and reduced daily use of rescue asthma medications.
Kauppi P et al. Sleep Breath. 2016 Dec;20(4):1217-1224.

☐
Treating moderate-severe OSA with CPAP improves lung function, asthma control and QOL in asthmatics. This prospective, multicenter study assessed asthma control (Asthma Control Questionnaire [ACQ]) and QOL (Mini Asthma Quality of Life Questionnaire (AQLQ)) in 99 adults with asthma and OSA (RDI ≥ 20) after 6 months of CPAP therapy. At 6 months, ACQ scores decreased significantly and AQLQ increased, along with reductions in the (a) percentage with uncontrolled asthma and (b) percentage with asthma attacks. Improvements in symptoms of GER and rhinitis, bronchial reversibility and exhaled nitric oxide values were observed. Drug therapy for asthma did not change.
Serrano-Pariente J et al. Allergy. 2016 Oct 12.

☐
Therapy with CPAP significantly lowers pulmonary artery pressure in OSA patients with pulmonary HTN. This article reported the meta-analysis results of 7 studies involving 222 patients with OSA (AHI > 10) whose pulmonary artery pressures were measured before and after CPAP

treatment (treatment duration of 3-70 months). Pulmonary HTN was defined as pulmonary artery pressure > 25 mmHg. The subjects had a mean age of 52.5 years, mean AHI of 58, and mean pulmonary artery pressure of 39.3 ± 6.3 mmHg. Using fixed effects meta-analysis, pulmonary artery pressure fell by 13.3 mmHg (95 % CI 12.7-14.0) was seen during CPAP therapy.

Imran TF et al. Heart Fail Rev. 2016 Sep;21(5):591-8.

☐

Presence and severity of OSA increases the risk of community-acquired pneumonia. A case control study compared the prevalence of OSA in 82 patients with community-acquired pneumonia (CAP) and 41 patients with non-respiratory infections (control). Subjects underwent respiratory polygraphy at the time of admission to the hospital, and the Pneumonia Severity Index was used to assess pneumonia severity. Obstructive sleep apnea (AHI ≥ 10) and OSA severity, based on AHI quartile, were both linked to CAP and CAP severity.

Chiner E et al. PLoS One. 2016 Apr 6;11(4):e0152749.

☐

Obstructive sleep apnea can cause acute pulmonary embolism. Results from a prospective cohort study showed that acute manifestations of pulmonary embolism were significantly more often to be sleep-related (i.e., caused an arousal from sleep or occurred within the 1st hour after waking) in patients with moderate-severe OSA compared to subjects with AHI ≤ 15. In 206 patients evaluated with portable monitoring and PSG, the risk of sleep-related acute pulmonary embolism increased relative to OSA severity.

Berghaus TM et al. Clin Res Cardiol. 2016 Jun 16.

☐

Obstructive sleep apnea is a risk factor for recurrent pulmonary embolism. Home respiratory polygraphy was recorded in 120 patients following discontinuation of oral anticoagulant therapy for a first episode of pulmonary embolism. Patients were followed for 5-8 years. During this time, pulmonary embolism recurred in 19 patients, and AHI was ≥ 10 in 16 of these patients. In a multivariate Cox regression model, independent risk factors for recurrent pulmonary embolism included AHI ≥ 10, mean nocturnal time with SaO_2, < 90% and D-dimer level. Independent risk factors for the resumption of oral anticoagulation therapy for a new thromboembolic event were AHI ≥ 10, mean nocturnal SaO_2, and ESS.

Alonso-Fernández A et al. Chest. 2016 Dec;150(6):1291-1301.

☐

Gastroesophaeal reflux is independently associated with OSA. Researchers conducted a multivariate cross-sectional analysis using a national database of ambulatory visits (National Ambulatory Medical Care Survey and National Hospital Ambulatory Medical Care Survey, 2005-2010). After adjustment for confounding factors, including age, gender, obesity, asthma and sinonasal, laryngopharyngeal and lung disorders, a significant positive association between GER and OSA was noted among adults.

Gilani S et al. Otolaryngol Head Neck Surg. 2016 Feb;154(2):390-5.

☐

Symptomatic nocturnal GER is common among patients with OSA, and CPAP ameliorates symptoms of nocturnal reflux. Seventy-eight percent (62 of 79) of patients complained of nocturnal GER symptoms during their initial visit. Nocturnal GER score correlated with sleep efficiency at baseline. Nocturnal GER score, ESS and CPAP compliance were reassessed at 6-month follow-up. Both nocturnal GER and ESS improved significantly in all patients at 6 months, but greater improvements were seen in CPAP-compliant patients. The authors noted that a CPAP compliance of ≥ 25% was required in order to achieve any benefit in noctural GER symptoms.

Tamanna S et al. J Clin Sleep Med. 2016 Sep 15;12(9):1257-61.

☐

Continuous positive airway pressure therapy does not cause GER in patients with moderate-severe OSA. Lower esophageal sphincter pressures, DeMeester scores and PSG parameters were evaluated pre- and post-CPAP in 25 patients with OSA (RDI > 15) who had no reflux symptoms. No significant differences were found between pre-CPAP and post-CPAP in either mean sphincter pressures (22.2 ± 1.2 vs. 22.9 ± 1.6) or mean DeMeester scores (18 ± 15.5 vs. 16.3 ± 14.8).

Ozcelik H et al. Eur Arch Otorhinolaryngol. 2016 Jun 22.

☐

Risk of liver injury increases in parallel with the severity of OSA. A cross-sectional study of 1,285 patients with suspected OSA assessed the relationship between the disorder and liver damage, including steatosis (hepatic steatosis index), cytolysis (alanine aminotransferase) and fibrosis (FibroMeter NAFLD score). Risk of liver steatosis increased with OSA severity and sleep-related hypoxemia (mean SaO_2) even after adjusting for confounders. A higher likelihood of liver cytolysis correlated with decreasing mean SaO_2 during sleep. Persons with severe OSA had a 2.5-fold increased risk for liver fibrosis compared to those without OSA; however, this association was not retained after adjustment for cofounding factors.

Trzepizur W et al. Clin Gastroenterol Hepatol. 2016 May 4.

☐

Biomarkers of liver damage are increased in untreated OSA and are not improved by 6-12 weeks of effective CPAP therapy. Three sham-controlled RCTs examined the effect of CPAP treatment on the FibroMax test in 103 patients with OSA (AHI > 15). Liver steatosis and borderline or possible non-alcoholic steatohepatitis (NASH) were present at baseline in 40% and 39.6% of sham-CPAP subjects, and 45% and 58.4% of CPAP subjects, respectively. Using CPAP for 6-12 weeks did not reduce steatosis, NASH or liver fibrosis.

Jullian-Desayes I et al. Respirology. 2016 Feb;21(2):378-85.

☐

In patients with OSA, CPAP therapy reduces the incidence, and delays the progression, of liver disease. This is a nationwide retrospective, population-based cohort study that evaluated the effects of CPAP treatment on liver disease in patients with OSA. Investigators used the Taiwan National Health Insurance claims database on CPAP and non-CPAP treated patients. Cumulative incidence rate of liver disease was lower in patients using CPAP compared to the non-CPAP group, and the risk of developing liver disease was lower in the CPAP group after adjusting for age, gender, level of urbanization and comorbidities.

Hang LW et al. Sleep Breath. 2016 Dec 13.

☐

Continuous positive airway pressure improves liver enzyme levels in OSA patients. A meta-analysis of 5 studies (seven cohorts of 192 patients) reported data on serum levels of alanine aminotransferase (ALT) and aspartate aminotransferase (AST) pre- and post-CPAP treatment. Levels of ALT and AST levels fell during CPAP therapy, especially if duration of therapy was > 3 months.
Chen LD et al. Clin Respir J. 2016 Sep 10.

☐

Prevalence of epilepsy is higher in OSA patients, and CPAP treatment reduces seizures. Prevalence of OSA was 33.4%, and was not affected by refractoriness, seizure type or number of anti-seizure drugs. Patients treated with CPAP had better seizure control than non-CPAP treated patients.
Lin Z et al. Sleep Breath. 2016 Jul 30.

☐

Obstructive sleep apnea is common in patients with late-onset epilepsy, and CPAP therapy reduces seizure frequency. Berlin Questionnaire, ESS and PSG were performed on 27 patients with late-onset epilepsy. Obstructive sleep apnea was present in 88.9% of the patients, who were then classified into no-mild OSA or moderate-severe OSA (55.6%). No significant inter-group differences were seen in EDS, CV risk factors, nocturnal seizure frequency, BMI or neck circumference. Patients with moderate-severe OSA were older. Frequency of seizures decreased in 80% of the patients who were given CPAP therapy.
Maurousset A et al. Neurophysiol Clin. 2016 Dec 14.

☐

Comorbid OSA worsens the prognosis of patients with ALS. Forty two patients with ALS were enrolled in a longitudinal retrospective study. Subjects were divided into OSA (AHI ≥ 5) and non-OSA (AHI < 5) groups. Mean survival was significantly shorter in the OSA group compared to controls. The authors noted significant correlations between the sniff nasal inspiratory pressure test and obstructive AHI, time with $SaO_2 < 90\%$ and ODI.
Quaranta VN et al. Neurodegener Dis. 2017;17(1):14-21.

☐
Polygraphy can predict respiratory failure and the need for NIV in patients with ALS with normal lung function. In this retrospective study, 131 patients with ALS underwent spirometry, nocturnal polygraphy and nocturnal ABG measurement. Nocturnal hypoventilation was identified in 67% of patients and was independent of their revised ALS-Functional Rating Scale (ALSFRS-R). Compared with the group that had normal nighttime ventilation, those with nocturnal hypoventilation had significantly lower vital capacity, FVC and maximal static inspiratory pressure.
Prell T et al. J Neurol Neurosurg Psychiatry. 2016 Mar 24.

☐
Using CPAP improves memory in patients with OSA. Memory, intellect and attention (Luria-Nebraska neuropsychological battery) were analyzed in 60 subjects, including 30 patients with OSA and 30 non-OSA controls. Areas of cognition were related to specific OSA parameters – between AHI and immediate memory, logical memory and thematic drawings, and between SaO_2 and immediate memory and thematic drawings. Using CPAP improved immediate memory in OSA patients.
Jurádo-Gámez B et al. Neurologia. 2016 Jun;31(5):311-318.

☐
A history of sleep apnea increases the risk of mood disorders. A population-based cohort, using data from the National Health Insurance database, assessed the likelihood of mood disorders in 5,415 patients with a history of sleep apnea and 27,075 matched non-sleep apnea controls. Mood disorder was diagnosed in 2.84% of patients with sleep apnea and in 1.13% of controls during the follow-up period. Sleep apnea was associated with a 1.82-2.07-fold greater risk of mood disorder than non-sleep apnea. Risk was highest for major depressive disorder and bipolar disorder and less for unspecified mood disorder.
Lu MK et al. Sleep Breath. 2016 Aug 5.

☐
There is a bidirectional causal relationship between OSA and depression. Researchers, using the Taiwan National Health Insurance Research Database, reported an association between OSA and depression. The study looked at 6,427 OSA patients and 32,135 controls,

and 27,073 patients with depression and 135,365 controls. Patients with OSA had an increased risk of future depression, and patients with depression had an increased risk of developing OSA after adjusting for potential confounders.

Pan ML et al. Medicine (Baltimore). 2016 Sep;95(37):e4833.

☐

Severity of EDS, but not AHI or O$_2$ desaturation, is linked to new-onset depression in patients with OSA. Adults without depression from the Penn State Adult Cohort (n = 1,137) underwent PSG at baseline and were followed-up after 7.5 years. Isolated OSA was not associated with incident depression but ESS, obesity (BMI ≥ 30) and being overweight (BMI 25-29.9) were, especially among 20-40 year old women.

LaGrotte C et al. Int J Obes (Lond). 2016 May 4.

☐

Treating OSA with PAP decreases PTSD symptoms in patients who have both disorders. In this prospective study, 59 patients with PTSD and newly diagnosed, untreated OSA were assessed at 3 and 6 months. Using CPAP significantly improved symptoms of PTSD (measured by PCL-S score), depression, sleep quality, sleepiness, daytime functioning, and QOL. Symptom improvement was related to % nights of PAP use, but not to mean hours of use per night.

Orr JE et al. J Clin Sleep Med. 2016 Sep 29.

☐
Upper airway collapsibility and pharyngeal dilator muscle activity vary in the different sleep stages. Passive pharyngeal critical closing pressure (Pcrit), a measure of UA collapsibility, was measured in 72 adults with and without OSA during periods of N2, SWS and REM sleep when CPAP settings were transiently reduced. Genioglossus and tensor palatini muscle activity were measured during wakefulness with and without CPAP, stable sleep on CPAP, and transient CPAP reductions. Collapsibility of the UA increased progressively during SWS, N2 and REM sleep. Muscle activity in the genioglossus, but not tensor palatini, decreased progressively from wakefulness to SWS, N2 and REM sleep.
Carberry JC et al. Sleep 2016. Sleep. 2016 Mar 1;39(3):511-21.

☐
Reduced stage N3 sleep is associated with many of the clinical symptoms seen in adult patients with OSA. In 30 adult subjects with OSA, excessive fatigue and waking up tired, sleepiness and falling asleep during the day, trouble paying attention, snoring and insomnia were significantly related to decreased stage N3 sleep.
Basunia M et al. J Community Hosp Intern Med Perspect. 2016 Sep 7;6(4):32170.

☐
Patients with OSA have shorter telomere lengths, a marker of cellular senescence. Leukocyte telomere length was measured using quantitative real-time polymerase chain reaction in 928 persons. Telomere length was significantly shorter in patients with OSA compared to controls. Telomere length was negatively correlated with AHI, RDI, ODI and WASO, and positively correlated with SE, TST, and basal, minimum and maximum SaO_2. After adjusting for sex, age, years of schooling, BMI, DM, stroke and heart attack, the severity of OSA was independently linked to shorter leukocyte telomere length.
Tempaku PF et al. Oncotarget. 2016 Sep 27.

☐
Intermittent hypoxemia related to OSA plays a role in telomere shortening in middle-aged men. Middle-aged men (n = 161) without

known comorbidities and who were CPAP-naïve were prospectively enrolled in this cross-sectional study. Obstructive sleep apnea was diagnosed using PSG. Patients with OSA had significantly shorter mean telomere length ratio compared to those without OSA. Telomere length was associated with ODI in multivariate analysis and negatively correlated with arterial stiffness as assessed by carotid-femoral pulse wave velocity.

Boyer L et al. Ann Am Thorac Soc. 2016 Jul;13(7):1136-43.

☐
Cumulative hypoxemia during sleep contributes more to vascular endothelial dysfunction in patients with SDB than does the frequency of hypoxemic events (e.g., AHI). The authors performed PSG and measured flow-mediated vasodilation response (%FMD) in 50 patients with suspected SDB. The %FMD had a significant relationship with averaged time desaturation summation index ([100%-averaged SaO_2] × TST) after adjusting for confounding factors, but not with AHI, 3% ODI, mean SaO_2, SaO_2min and ratio of SaO_2 < 90%.

Sawatari H et al. Am J Hypertens. 2016 Apr;29(4):458-63.

☐
Impairment of physical functioning and EDS in patients with OSA are related to duration and severity of O_2 desaturation rather than to AHI or measures of sleep architecture. Polysomnography was performed on, and ESS and SF-36 questionnaires were completed by, 88 patients. Polysomnography parameters correlated with Physical Function, Physical Component Summary and ESS. The OSA group (≥ 5) had significantly lower scores on 7 SF-36 domains. Physical Function and Physical Component Summary, but not ESS scores, worsened as AHI increased. In multiple linear regression analysis, only measures of O_2 desaturation were significant predictors of Physical Function and ESS. Physical Function decreased by 0.59 points and ESS increased by 0.13 points for every 1% fall in SaO_2min.

Huang W et al. Ann Acad Med Singapore. 2016 Sep;45(9):404-412.

☐
Intermittent hypoxia related to OSA is associated with LV hypertrophy in persons with well-controlled HTN. This cross-sectional study enrolled 223 men with HTN, sleep apnea and normal cardiac function. Subjects

underwent PSG and echocardiography. Left ventricular mass index correlated significantly with the integrated area of desaturation (IAD), a marker of intermittent hypoxia, but not with AHI. Independent variables affecting the LV mass index included IAD, BNP and age.

Yamaguchi T et al. Am J Hypertens. 2016 Mar;29(3):372-8.

☐

Endocan, a marker of endothelial dysfunction, is elevated in patients with OSA. Flow-mediated dilatation (FMD), carotid intima media thickness (CIMT) and serum endocan levels were measured in 40 subjects with OSA at baseline and after 3 months of CPAP treatment, and in 40 controls. Endocan was a good predictor of OSA, with its levels being significantly higher in subjects with OSA than in controls. Endocan levels correlated with AHI, and levels decreased significantly after 3 months of CPAP treatment. Both endocan levels and AHI were significantly and independently correlated with CIMT and FMD.

Altintas N et al. Angiology. 2016 Apr;67(4):364-74.

☐

Serum level of endocan, a marker for premature vascular endothelial cell injury, is higher in patients with OSA compared to healthy individuals. This is a cohort study that consisted of 113 patients with OSA (AHI ≥ 5) and 15 controls. Both flow-mediated dilatation (FMD) and plasma endocan levels were measured to assess endothelial function. Compared to healthy controls, patients with OSA had significantly higher endocan levels and lower FMD measures. The AHI was positively correlated with serum endocan levels and negatively correlated with FMD.

Kanbay A et al. Clin Respir J. 2016 Apr 26.

☐

Long-term CPAP therapy has beneficial effects on antioxidant capacity and cardiovascular risk biomarkers, but not glucose homeostasis or insulin sensitivity, in non-obese, non-diabetic patients with OSA. Oral glucose tolerance, insulin sensitivity, oxidative stress and CV biomarkers were measured before and after long-term CPAP use (13.9 ± 6.5 months) in 28 patients with OSA. Insulin resistance was associated with nocturnal O_2 desaturation. Long-term treatment with CPAP increased plasma total antioxidant status, decreased homocysteine and NT-proBNP levels, but

had no effect on oral glucose tolerance.
Monneret D et al. Respir Med. 2016 Mar;112:119-25.

☐
Objective EDS, but not subjective EDS, is associated with elevated IL-6 and decreased daytime cortisol levels in patients with OSA. Daytime sleepiness was measured objectively with MSLT, and subjectively using ESS and Stanford Sleepiness Scale (SSS) in 58 patients with OSA who underwent PSG for 4 consecutive nights. Twenty-four hour profiles of IL-6 and cortisol levels were measured on the 4th day. Levels of IL-6 (24-hour, daytime and nighttime) were elevated and daytime cortisol levels were significantly lower in patients with documented objective sleepiness. These changes in IL-6 or cortisol levels were not linked to subjective EDS.
Li Y et al. Sleep. 2016 Oct 10.

☐
Increased caloric intake predicts weight gain in OSA patients using CPAP. To better understand why some OSA patients gain weight while using CPAP, researchers measured energy metabolism in 63 patients with newly diagnosed OSA at baseline, at CPAP initiation and at 3-month follow-up. Whereas basal metabolic rate decreased significantly after CPAP was started, physical activity and total caloric intake were unchanged. Patients who gained weight had higher leptin levels and lower ghrelin levels than non-weight gainers. Disordered eating behavior, including increased caloric intake, was more common in those who gained weight.
Tachikawa R et al. Am J Respir Crit Care Med. 2016 Mar 1.

☐

Colonization of the tonsils by group A streptococcus might play a role in the pathogenesis of pediatric OSA. A significant association between group A streptococcus (GAS) and OSA was found in 40 tonsillectomized children. Streptolysin-O from GAS may induce the production of cysteinyl leukotrienes by tonsillar mononuclear cells and give rise to tonsillar hyperplasia.
Viciani E et al. Sci Rep. 2016 Feb 10;6:20609.

☐

There is a tendency for OSA to resolve in prepubertal children as they transition to adolescence. In this longitudinal study, 421 of 700 elementary school children were assessed at baseline and were reevaluated during adolescence 8 years later (Penn State Child Cohort). Remission to AHI ≥ 2 and ≥ 5 were seen in 52.9% and 100.0% of children, respectively. Primary snoring and mild SDB do not generally progress to more severe disease. Main risk factors for adolescent SDB were male gender, age and obesity.
Bixler EO et al. Eur Respir J. 2016 Feb 4.

☐

Psychosocial dysfunction persists despite resolution of SDB in children. Polysomnography was repeated at 6-8 years in children, aged 3-5 years, with snoring or OSA, and in healthy non-snoring controls. Resolution, whether spontaneous or following treatment, was defined as an OAHI ≤ 1 or absence of snoring, and was seen in only 50% of snorers, 45% of children with mild OSA and 63% of those with moderate-severe OSA. Improvements in physical symptoms, school functioning, and family worry and relationships were seen with reduced OAHI.
Biggs SN et al. J Pediatr. 2015 Dec;167(6):1272-1279.e1.

☐

Obesity during childhood heightens the risk of OSA developing during middle age. About 23.9% of children were noted to be overweight at initial assessment in the Bogalusa Heart Study. After 35 years of follow-up, 25.7% had BQ scores indicating a high risk for OSA (positive score in ≥ 2 domains with obesity removed from scoring). Subjects with persistent

51

and incident excess weight were 1.36 and 1.47 times more likely to be high risk for OSA compared to those who were never overweight.
Bazzano LA et al. Pediatr Obes. 2016 Jan 19.

☐
Obstructive sleep apnea is linked to metabolic derangements in obese adolescents. This literature review included 16 articles in a qualitative synthesis and 10 in a meta-analysis. The meta-analysis revealed that the presence of OSA in adolescents increased the likelihood of HTN, dyslipidemia and insulin resistance.
Patinkin ZW et al. Child Obes. 2016 Dec 12.

☐
In children with OSA, the presence and severity of insulin resistance are increased by obesity. Investigators reported that higher AHIs were associated with greater insulin resistance among 459 children (5-12 years of age). Glucose levels and insulin resistance were inversely correlated with sleep duration (N3 and REM sleep) and positively associated with sleep fragmentation.
Koren D et al. Eur Respir J. 2016 Feb 4.

☐
Moderate-severe OSA has a deleterious effect on neurocognitive functioning in young school-aged children. Investigators prospectively performed PSG and neurocognitive assessments of intellectual, attention, memory, language, and executive function in 1,010 snoring and non-snoring children aged 5-7 years. There was a dose-response impact of SDB, and those with severe OSA (AHI >5) were significantly more impaired than groups with less severe AHIs in Differential Ability Scales Verbal and Nonverbal performance, and global conceptual ability. Subscores on specific NEPSY, a developmental neuropsychological assessment that focuses on attention and executive skills, also differed across groups.
Hunter SJ et al. Am J Respir Crit Care Med. 2016 Sep 15;194(6):739-47.

☐
Adenotonsillectomy improves OSA in most children. However, a high risk of residual OSA (AHI > 2) was noted in teenagers and children with severe OSA, obesity, asthma and comorbidities (neurological,

developmental or craniofacial abnormalities). This is a retrospective chart review of 169 children with OSA who underwent AT. Prevalence of residual OSA was 38% (overall), 49% (obese), 27% (non-obese), 44% (neurological, developmental or craniofacial abnormalities), 33% (without comorbidities), 42% (severe OSA), 29% (moderate OSA), 0% (mild OSA), 67% (teenagers), 27% (toddlers), 33% (preschoolers), and 29% (middle childhood group).

Imanguli M et al. Laryngoscope. 2016 Nov;126(11):2624-2629.

☐
Adenotonsillectomy, as therapy for OSA, is less effective in obese children than in normal-weight children. Investigators reviewed 16 articles that dealt with outcomes of OSA therapy in obese children and adolescents. Obstructive sleep apnea was significantly more likely to persist in obese children after AT. The prevalence of persistent OSA after AT was 33-76% in obese children and 15-37% in non-obese children. In comparison, the prevalence of persistent OSA was 10-38% after weight loss. Although PAP was an effective therapy, 2 of 3 studies reported a mean nightly use of < 4 hours.

Andersen IG et al. Int J Pediatr Otorhinolaryngol. 2016 Aug;87:190-7.

☐
Montelukast, a leukotriene inhibitor, reduces the severity of OSA in children 2-10 years of age. This is a double-blind, randomized, placebo-controlled trial that involved 64 children with OSA who were given oral montelukast (4 or 5 mg daily) or placebo for 16 weeks. The two groups were matched for age, gender, initial AHI and percentage of obesity. Eighty-nine percent of the subjects completed the trial. Automated timed pill dispensers and weekly telephonic reminders were used to ascertain medication adherence. Significantly more children who received montelukast experienced a reduction in AHI compared to the placebo group (71.4% vs. 6.9%). In montelukast-treated children, AHI decreased significantly from 9.2 ± 4.1 to 4.2 ± 2.8.

Kheirandish-Gozal L et al. Ann Am Thorac Soc. 2016 Oct;13(10):1736-1741.

☐
Pregnant women with chronic disease, especially HTN and DM, have a higher likelihood of OSA compared to healthy pregnant women. Questionnaires, including BQ, ESS, socio-demographic information and pregnancy characteristics were completed by 97 pregnant women with chronic diseases and 160 healthy pregnant women. A high risk of OSA was noted in 20.6-23.3% of all pregnant women, and was more common in those with chronic diseases than in healthy women (34-45.4% vs. 10-12.5%, respectively).
Karaduman M et al. J Matern Fetal Neonatal Med. 2016 Oct;29(20):3379-85.

☐
The likelihood of preterm delivery is increased in pregnant women who have a high risk of OSA. Screening for OSA during the second trimester of pregnancy using BQ was performed in this prospective cohort study of 1,345 pregnant women. Prevalence of high-risk OSA was 10.1%, and the adjusted odds ratio for preterm delivery in this group was 2.00 (95% CI 1.20, 3.34). High-risk OSA was associated with an increased risk of spontaneous preterm delivery after adjusting for confounding factors.
Na-Rungsri K et al. Sleep Breath. 2016 Sep;20(3):1111-7.

☐
Maternal SDB can result in delivery of small-for-gestational-age infants. A prospective cohort study enrolled 234 pregnant women who had PSG-based diagnosis of SDB in their third trimester. Overall sensitivity and specificity of symptoms were both poor for PSG-diagnosed SDB. Twelve percent of participants delivered small-for-gestational-age (< 10th centile) infants. An AHI threshold of 10 significantly increased the odds of delivering a small-for-gestational-age infant.
Pamidi S et al. Thorax. 2016 Apr 15.

☐
Each additional year in menopause increases AHI by 4%. This change was independent of aging and changes in body habitus according to the Sleep in Midlife Women Study. Using longitudinal data on sleep, including in-home PSG studies every 6 months, and menopausal health metrics

from 219 participants in the Wisconsin Sleep Cohort Study, AHIs were noted to be 21% higher during peri-menopause and 31% higher in post-menopause compared to pre-menopause.
Mirer AG et al. Menopause. 2016 Oct 10.

☐
Several OSA risk factors are associated with nocturnal enuresis in postmenopausal women. A cross-sectional study of 2,789 women aged 50 to 79 years (Women's Health Initiative Observational Study) reported a 1.7% prevalence of nocturnal enuresis. Factors associated with nocturnal enuresis included daytime sleepiness, HTN, obesity, poor sleep quality, sleep fragmentation and snoring, and each additional risk factor increased, in a dose response manner, the odds of nocturnal enuresis .
Koo P et al. Menopause. 2016 Feb;23(2):175-82.

☐
Three months of CPAP therapy improves QOL, mood and daytime sleepiness in women with moderate-severe OSA. This is a multicenter, open-label RCT involving women (n = 307 in 19 sleep units; mean age of 57.1 ± 10.1 years; mean ESS score of 9.8 ± 4.4; 77.5% postmenopausal) with moderate-severe OSA (AHI ≥ 15). Subjects were randomized to effective CPAP therapy or conservative treatment for 3 months. The CPAP group had significantly greater improvements in all QOL domains of the Quebec Sleep Questionnaire, daytime sleepiness, mood state, anxiety, depression, and the physical component of the 12-item Short Form Health Survey compared to controls.
Campos-Rodriguez F et al. Am J Respir Crit Care Med. 2016 Nov 15;194(10):1286-1294.

☐

Older adults have a higher prevalence of OSA and more severe disease compared to younger patients. In addition, elderly patients (≥ 65 years) had worse sleep quality, more severe nocturnal O_2 desaturation, and higher percentages of HTN, CAD and arrhythmias versus younger patients. However, odds ratio for HTN increased with OSA severity only in younger patients.
Hua-Huy T et al. Aging Clin Exp Res. 2015 Oct;27(5):611-9.

☐

Aging increases OSA severity in older adults. Forty four non-elderly adults (aged < 65 years) and 46 elderly adults (aged ≥ 65 years) were divided into mild-moderate OSA (5 < AHI < 30) and severe OSA (AHI ≥ 30) groups. The severe OSA group was older and had higher BMI than the mild-moderate group among older adults. Age was correlated with AHI only in older adults. There were no significant differences between mild-moderate OSA and severe OSA in older adults in terms of physical strength, cognitive function, apathy scale, depression scale or activities of daily living.
Hongyo K et al. Geriatr Gerontol Int. 2016 Jun 1.

☐

Healthy older adults with SDB have greater cognitive decline. The PROOF cohort followed 559 adults without neurological disorders for 8 years. At baseline, SDB (AHI > 15) was present in 54% of subjects, and severe SDB ((AHI > 30) in 18%. A significant decline in attentional and memory function was observed in patients with SDB, and the degree of decline in attention was related to AHI, whereas the decline in memory correlated with sleep fragmentation.
Martin MS et al. Ann Phys Rehabil Med. 2016 Sep;59S:e99.

☐

Older men with obstructive airway disease are less likely to develop sleep apnea. Data on sleep (using home PSG) and lung function (based on spirometry) from the Outcomes of Sleep Disorders in Older Men Study, which involved 853 community-dwelling older men, identified obstructive airway disease (pre-bronchodilator FEV_1/FVC ratio < 0.7 and FEV_1 < 80%

predicted) and sleep apnea (AHI ≥ 15) in 13.0% and 29.0% of the men, respectively. Subjects with obstructive airway disease had lower AHIs as well as a lower prevalence of sleep apnea compared to those without obstructive airway disease. The group with comorbid obstructive airway disease and sleep apnea had increased arousal indices and lower SaO_2 levels vs. subjects with isolated obstructive airway disease.

Zhao YY et al. Sleep. 2016 Apr 12.

☐

Long-term use of CPAP reduces the frequency and duration of napping in older adults with OSA. This retrospective cohort study involved 107 adults aged ≥ 60 years with OSA who were started on CPAP treatment. Subjects with a history of stroke or CV disease had more frequent napping before initiating CPAP treatment. Duration of CPAP treatment was 82.7 ± 30.0 weeks and objective adherence was 5.4 ± 2.0 hours per night. Significantly less daytime and evening napping, and shorter daily nap duration were reported during CPAP use.

Hsieh CF et al. J Am Geriatr Soc. 2016 Jun 30.

☐

About half of anesthesiologists rely on clinical suspicion alone to identify undiagnosed OSA preoperatively rather than using a systematic screening protocol. A scenario-based questionnaire survey of Canadian anesthesiologists also revealed that 47% of respondents were not aware of any institutional policy that dealt with the perioperative management of OSA patients.

Cordovani L et al. Can J Anaesth. 2015 Oct 19.

☐

STOP-Bang is a reliable screening tool for OSA. A meta-analysis of 17 studies, which included 9,206 patients, showed that the probability of severe OSA with a STOP-Bang score of 3 was 25% and 15% in the sleep clinic and surgical populations, respectively. The probability increased in a stepwise fashion with higher STOP-Bang scores. Sensitivity in moderate-severe OSA (AHI ≥ 15) was 94%.

Nagappa M et al. PLoS One. 2015 Dec 14;10(12):e0143697.

☐

The STOP-Bang screening questionnaire is better at detecting OSA than STOP, BQ and ESS questionnaires. In a bivariate meta-analysis, investigators compared the sensitivity, specificity and diagnostic odds ratio (DOR) of the 4 screening tools in 108 studies that included 47,989 participants. Pooled sensitivity and DOR of STOP-Bang were significantly higher than the other questionnaires, but its specificity was lower than that of ESS.

Chiu HY et al. Sleep Med Rev. 2016 Nov 5.

☐

The STOP-Bang questionnaire can help identify which obese patients with OSA have coexisting OHS. This study included 105 subjects with OSA, 196 who were obese, and 74 with OHS and OSA. Both the original and modified versions of the STOP-Bang questionnaire scores were higher in the OHS group than in the pure OSA group. In the modified STOP-Bang questionnaire, BMI was divided into ranges and serum bicarbonate levels were considered. An original STOP-Bang questionnaire score of ≥ 6 and the modified STOP-Bang questionnaire had sensitivities of 71.6% and 89.2%; specificities of 59.1% and 47.6%; PPV of 55.2% and 54.6%; and NPV of 74.7% and 86.2%, respectively.

Bingol Z et al. Sleep Breath. 2016 May;20(2):495-500.

☐

The Sleep Apnea Clinical Score reliably detects OSA in primary care medical patients. In this prospective cohort study, Sleep Apnea Clinical Score (SACS) testing, overnight oximetry and PSG were performed on 312 adult family medicine patients. A SACS score > 15 was 40% sensitive and 90% specific in identifying OSA (AHI > 10), with a PPV of 73% and a NPV of 69%.

Grover M et al. Mayo Clin Proc. 2016 Mar 5.

☐

Neither ESS nor BQ are adequately accurate in driving candidates for OSA. In this population, ESS had a low sensitivity and BQ suffered from a low specificity. This study enrolled 223 patients suspected of having OSA. Questionnaires (ESS and BQ) and PSG were conducted to differentiate persons with no or mild OSA (AHI < 15) vs. those with moderate-severe OSA (AHI ≥ 15). Sensitivity of 53.2% and 93.1%, and specificity of 58.8% and 16.2% were noted for ESS and BQ, respectively. Correlation between the ESS score and AHI and AI was poor.

Kiciński P et al. Med Pr. 2016 Dec 22;67(6):721-728.

☐

The BQ and ESS perform poorly as screening questionnaires for OSA in pregnant women. Six articles were included in this meta-analysis. The pooled prevalence of OSA during pregnancy was 26.7%. Pooled sensitivity and specificity of ESS were poor at 0.44 and 0.62, respectively. Performance of BQ was only slightly better with a pooled sensitivity of 0.66 and a specificity of 0.62. Sensitivity of BQ was lower during early pregnancy (≤ 20 weeks gestation) and in high-risk pregnancies.

Tantrakul V et al. Sleep Med Rev. 2016 Nov 15.

☐

Oximetry is a useful screening tool for identifying patients with severe OSA. Investigators prospectively studied 204 patients using home oximetry combined with 4 questionnaires, namely STOP, STOP-Bang, BQ and ESS, and in-laboratory PSG. Oximetry and PSG were performed within 3-20 days of each other. Oximetry had a high predictive value for severe, but not mild-moderate, OSA. Combining oximetry with the various questionnaires did not improve diagnostic predictive accuracy for mild-moderate OSA. Of the 4 questionnaires, STOP-Bang had the highest sensitivity and NPV (97.5% and 62.5%, respectively) and the lowest specificity (9%). The ESS has the best specificity and PPV (75% and 81.4%, respectively).

Pataka A et al. Ann Transl Med. 2016 Nov;4(22):443.

☐

A two-step screening strategy can effectively identify OSA in healthy workers. Investigators enrolled 1,861 employees in a cross-sectional study using a new questionnaire. Subjects subsequently underwent nasal flow recording and home PSG on two separate nights. Data from nasal flow and PSG were available for 71% of the subjects. Among these, OSA was diagnosed in 36.9%. Obstructive sleep apnea was best predicted by a combination of age, absence of insomnia, witnessed apneas, and Berlin and STOP-Bang questionnaires. A new questionnaire was constructed and, along with nasal flow recording, had a high sensitivity (63.1%) and specificity (90.1%).

Eijsvogel MM et al. J Clin Sleep Med. 2016 Apr 15.

☐

Demographic and PSG parameters can be used to estimate cardiovascular disease in patients with SDB. Researchers conducted a retrospective review of clinical and PSG data from 1,162 consecutive patients with suspected SDB, of whom 20.1% had a history of CV disease. Nineteen parameters were associated with CV disease, including age (most important), TST with $SaO_2 < 90\%$, SaO_2min, AHI during NREM, BMI, SDB severity, and total, mean and longest apnea duration. Using Bayesian network analysis, a final model was created with a sensitivity, specificity and NPV of 76.9%, 96.2% and 92.6%, respectively.
Turhan M et al. Eur Arch Otorhinolaryngol. 2016 Jun 30.

☐

Certain oropharyngeal examination features (e.g., tongue indentations and tonsillar grades III and IV) are associated with risk of OSA. In this cross-sectional study, 200 dental patients were evaluated for habitual snoring and OSA risk using BQ. An estimated 82% of men and 18% of women reported habitual snoring, and high-risk of OSA was noted in about 78% and 22% of men and women, respectively. Obesity, tongue indentations, tonsil size and sleepiness were independent risk factors for OSA.
Al-Jewair TS et al. Saudi Med J. 2016 Feb;37(2):183-90.

☐

A sawtooth sign in spirometry is predictive of OSA. Fifty subjects who demonstrated a sawtooth sign during spirometric examination and 100 controls matched for age, weight and gender were assessed for OSA. A diagnosis of OSA was present in 44% of subjects with a sawtooth sign compared to 27% of controls. After adjusting for age, weight, gender and pack years of smoking, the sawtooth sign remained an important risk for OSA. The authors commented that the sawtooth sign may be a marker of redundant UA tissue.
Bourne MH Jr et al. Sleep Breath. 2016 Nov 29.

☐

Several factors predict the presence of OSA on PSG after a normal HST in patients with a high pretest probability of the disease. In this

61

retrospective study, 24% and 71% of patients with normal (n = 127) or technically inadequate (n = 111) HSTs, respectively, had OSA on PSG testing. A normal PSG is more likely in patients < 50 years of age with a normal HST, whereas older age in persons with technically inadequate HSTs increased the likelihood of OSA being diagnosed during PSG.
Zeidler MR et al. J Clin Sleep Med. 2015 Nov 15;11(11):1313-8.

☐
Night-to-night variability in AHI during HST is more pronounced in mild OSA compared to moderate-severe OSA. In this prospective observational study, 84 patients with newly diagnosed OSA (AHI ≥ 5) by PSG underwent 2-8 consecutive nights of HST. Mean AHI on PSG and HST were 30.1 ± 31.8 and 27.4 ± 23.7, respectively. Night-to-night AHI variability was greater in those with mild OSA (AHI 5-15).
Prasad B et al. J Clin Sleep Med. 2016 Feb 1.

☐
Different definitions of hypopnea impact the prevalence and severity classification of OSA, and its associated cardiovascular outcomes in women and older adults. Three hypopnea definitions, namely a 30-90% reduction in oronasal flow for ≥ 10 s associated with (a) ≥ 4% fall in SaO_2 [AHI4%], (b) ≥ 3% fall in SaO_2 [AHI3%] or (c) ≥ 3% fall in SaO_2 or an event-related arousal [AHI3%/A], were analyzed in 1,116 women and 939 elderly individuals. Using the AHI3%/A criterion increased the prevalence of OSA (AHI ≥ 30) by 14% with compared with AHI4%. An AHI ≥ 30 was associated with increased risk of CV mortality in women (regardless of the definition of hypopnea used) and in elderly individuals (when AHI4% and AHI3%, but not AHI3%/A, definitions were used) in fully adjusted multivariable analyses.
Campos-Rodriguez F et al. Sleep Med. 2016 Nov - Dec; 27-28:54-58.

☐
Fewer younger patients are eligible for CPAP therapy if CMS, rather than AASM, criteria are used. Differences in PSG scoring rules for hypopneas between the AASM and Center for Medicare and Medicaid Services (CMS) were assessed in 112 consecutive patients. The rate of treatment eligibility was the same with either method in older Medicare-aged patients, but using the CMS criteria lowered scorable AHI in younger patients.

Korotinsky A et al. Sleep Breath. 2016 Mar 11.

☐
Modifications to the current diagnostic criteria for split-night PSG are needed for Asian patients. Researchers compared full-night PSG data with data from the first 2 hours of sleep in 134 patients with OSA (AHI ≥ 5). There was no difference in AHI noted between the two data sets. Compared to the current AASM criterion of AHI ≥ 40 in the first 2 hours to qualify for a split night study, the threshold of AHI ≥ 30 had a better diagnostic accuracy and higher correlation with full night data.
Kim DK et al. Sleep Breath. 2015 Dec;19(4):1273-7.

☐
This report describes the validation of the DES-OSA, a clinical score based solely on morphologic features. Morphologic metrics from 149 patients who underwent overnight PSGs were compared. Five variables with the best prediction abilities (Mallampati score, distance between the thyroid and the chin, BMI, neck circumference and sex) were weighted using 1, 2, or 3 points. Increased probability of an AHI > 5, > 15, or > 30 were associated with DES-OSA scores of > 5, 6 and 7, respectively.
Deflandre E et al. Anesth Analg. 2016 Feb;122(2):363-72.

☐
Chest wall EMG assists in the classification of apneas during PSG when used along with respiratory inductance plethysmography. Chest wall EMG, recorded from electrodes placed in the 8th intercostal space, right mid-axillary line, was compared to dual channel uncalibrated respiratory inductance plethysmography (RIP) in their accuracy to classify apneas as obstructive, central or mixed in 20 clinical sleep studies (4 obstructive and 6 central/mixed apnea). Percentage agreement between the 2 methods was 89.5%. Ten percent of apneas classified as central by RIP was reclassified as obstructive and 3% as mixed by chest wall EMG. Conversely, 3% of apneas classified as central by chest wall EMG was reclassified as obstructive and 3% as mixed by RIP.
Berry RB et al. J Clin Sleep Med. 2016 Jun 9.

☐
Metabolomic profiling distinguishes OSA from simple snoring and non-OSA. Metabolomics was used to analyze urinary metabolites in patients

with PSG-confirmed OSA, simple snorers and normal controls. Several metabolites were differentially expressed in the various groups. The combination of 4-hydroxypentenoic acid, arabinose, glycochenodeoxycholate-3-sulfate, isoleucine, serine, and xanthine was able to distinguish OSA from non-OSA with a sensitivity and specificity of 75% and 78%, respectively; whereas the combination of 4-hydroxypentenoic acid, 5-dihydrotestosterone sulfate, serine, spermine, and xanthine had a sensitivity and specificity of 85% and 80%, respectively, in differenting OSA from simple snoring.
Xu H et al. Sci Rep. 2016 Aug 2;6:30958.

☐
Acoustic pharyngometry provides no additional insights over clinical variables in diagnosing OSA. Acoustic pharyngometry is a technique that is used to assess UA cross-sectional area. In this cross-sectional study, PSG and acoustic pharyngometry were conducted in 576 subjects, 87% of whom had OSA (AHI ≥ 5). Patients with OSA had significantly smaller median UA cross-sectional area at functional residual capacity when sitting than non-OSA patients, and a cutoff value of 3.75 cm^2 had a sensitivity and specificity of 73% and 46%, respectively. The incremental discriminative value of this measure over clinical variables, such as age, sex, BMI, and comorbidities, was not significant.
Kendzerska T et al. Ann Am Thorac Soc. 2016 Nov;13(11):2019-2026.

☐
Implanted cardiac pacemakers can reliably detect the presence of OSA. A validated algorithm measured respiratory disturbances in 58 patients with implanted dual-chamber pacemakers. Mean RDI was 19.9 ± 12.7 and was > 20 in 41% of patients during a mean follow-up of 187 ± 123 days. Ninety percent of patients had at least one night with an RDI > 20. Mean day-to-day individual RDI variability was 19% ± 21%. An RDI > 20 correlated with severe OSA as determined by PSG. No RDI threshold was predictive of AF recurrence. A high burden of severe OSA (i.e., ≥ 75% of nights with RDI > 20) was associated with older age, higher prevalence of HTN and more implantation procedures for AV block.
Moubarak G et al. Heart Rhythm. 2016 Nov 23.

☐
Analysis of exhaled breath accurately detects OSA recurrence. Thirty

subjects with OSA, who were effectively treated with CPAP, were randomized to either subtherapeutic or therapeutic CPAP for 2 weeks. Twenty six subjects completed the study. Exhaled breath was analyzed using secondary-electrospray-ionization-mass spectrometry at baseline and after 2 weeks of randomization. Subtherapeutic CPAP was associated with recurrence of OSA as well as significant changes in several exhaled breath metrics, a panel of which differentiated treated and untreated OSA with a sensitivity and specificity of 92.9% and 84.6%, respectively.

Schwarz EI et al. Thorax. 2016 Feb;71(2):110-7.

☐
Treating mild OSA may improve sleepiness and QOL in sleepy persons.
The American Thoracic Society published its research statement on the
adverse CV and neurocognitive effects of mild OSA in adults. Evidence on
the relationship between mild OSA and EDS was variable. Data on the
effects of therapy on arrhythmias, CV events, mood, neurocognition,
stroke and car accidents were also limited or inconsistent.
Chowdhuri S et al. Am J Respir Crit Care Med. 2016 May 1;193(9):e37-54.

☐
**Management of sleep apnea using a telemedicine-based strategy is
cost-effective.** Similar CPAP compliance, improvements in daytime
sleepiness and QOL, adverse effects and patient satisfaction were found
at 6 months for standard face-to-face care vs. telemedicine in an RCT
involving 139 patients. Total costs were lower with telemedicine.
Isetta V et al. Thorax. 2015 Nov;70(11):1054-61.

☐
**Telemedicine increases the efficiency of administering sleep services to
patients with sleep apnea.** A 5-year U.S. Veterans Administration study
showed that a comprehensive sleep telemedicine protocol improved the
timeliness of interventions for sleep apnea despite an increase in the
number of services provided. Electronic consultation based on chart
review was used to determine the next step in intervention. Notably, the
waiting period from sleep consultation to PAP prescription fell from ≥ 60
days to ≤ 7 days, but there was no change in clinic wait time, which
remained at 60 days or more.
Baig MM et al. Telemed J E Health. 2016 Mar 14.

☐
**Telemonitoring of CPAP treatment reduces the time that patients with
OSA require nursing care.** After CPAP titration, 111 patients were
managed by usual care or via telemetry. Medical nursing time was
significantly shorter in the telemonitoring group than in the usual care
group. There was no difference in CPAP adherence between groups, and
residual AHI was marginally better in patients followed by
telemonitoring.

Anttalainen U et al. Sleep Breath. 2016 Dec;20(4):1209-1215.

☐

Adult patients with OSA who were unable to tolerate PAP therapy are unlikely to be referred for additional therapies. A retrospective review of 616 patients documented PAP adherence in 42%. Only 35% of untreated patients were referred for other treatments.
Russell JO et al. Otolaryngol Head Neck Surg. 2015 Nov;153(5):881-7.

☐

Morbid obesity, COPD and older age (> 50 years), but not HF, can lead to persistent hypoxia during PAP therapy for sleep apnea and result in unanticipated need for nocturnal O_2 supplementation. Two hundred patients with OSA were included in a retrospective study that examined the contributory role of medical comorbidities in persistent hypoxia during PAP therapy. Postural O_2 desaturation between upright and reclining positions during calm wakefulness was significantly more pronounced in patients who needed combined PAP and nocturnal O_2 therapy vs. the group that needed only PAP.
Shetty S et al. J Clin Sleep Med. 2016 Sep 13.

☐
Effective AHI, the sum of SDB events when PAP is used *plus* not used during the sleep period, may be high in patients with OSA who are not using their PAP device throughout the night. A prospective cohort study evaluated 28 adult patients who were prescribed CPAP therapy for OSA. Effective AHI is defined as apneas-hypopneas with PAP ON *plus* apneas-hypopneas with PAP OFF *divided by* TST. Mean AHI were 67.9 (diagnostic) and 18.3 (effective). All patients who used PAP ≥ 6 hours nightly had an effective-AHI < 5. In patients who used PAP < 6 hours, 63.6% had residual moderate-severe OSA.
Boyd SB et al. Sleep. 2016 Nov 1;39(11):1961-1972.

☐
Adding CPAP therapy to usual care significantly improves snoring, EDS, HRQOL and mood, but did not prevent cardiovascular events, in patients with moderate-severe OSA and cardiovascular disease compared with usual care alone. Patients with moderate-severe OSA (n = 2,717; aged 45-75 years) and a history of coronary or cerebrovascular disease were randomized to CPAP treatment plus usual care or usual care alone. Primary composite end point (death from CV causes, MI, stroke, or hospitalization for unstable angina, HF or TIA) and secondary end points (other CV outcomes, HRQOL, snoring, daytime sleepiness and mood) were measured. Adherence to CPAP therapy was 3.3 hours per night, and CPAP decreased AHI from 29.0 at baseline to 3.7 during a mean follow-up of 3.7 years. Occurrence of a primary end-point event did not significantly differ between the CPAP and usual care groups (17.0% and 15.4%, respectively). Therapy with CPAP did not significantly affect any single or composite CV end point.
McEvoy RD et al. N Engl J Med. 2016 Sep 8;375(10):919-31.

☐
Positive airway pressure therapy improves endotherlial function, arterial tone and diastolic function in young to middle-aged adults with OSA. These benefits depended on hours of use, were present after 4 weeks of treatment, but disappeared rapidly after withdrawal of therapy. In a prospective study, echocardiography and brachial artery reactivity testing were performed on 84 subjects (AHI 39.8 ± 24.5) at baseline, at 4

and 12 weeks of PAP therapy, and 1 week after PAP withdrawal. At 4 and 12 weeks, PAP therapy was associated with reductions in central systolic BP, diastolic BP, mean BP, aortic augmentation index, peripheral pulse wave velocity, and brachial artery dilation; and improved LV diastolic function, and systemic and pulmonary vascular resistance. Hours per night of PAP use predicted improvements in diastolic BP, aortic augmentation index, peripheral pulse wave velocity, and brachial artery flow-mediated dilation. Regrettably, improvements in brachial diameter, diastolic BP, mean BP, aortic augmentation index, and HR reversed after 1 week of PAP withdrawal.

Korcarz CE et al. J Am Heart Assoc. 2016 Apr 3;5(4).

☐

Changes in inflammatory markers observed in OSA, including nuclear factor-κβ, hypoxia-inducible factor-1 alpha and surfactant protein D protein, are reversed by CPAP therapy. Serum levels of inflammatory markers were measured in 25 patients with mild-moderate OSA, 33 patients with severe OSA, and 20 healthy patients (control group). Patients with severe OSA received CPAP therapy and were evaluated after 2 months. Expression of nuclear factor-κβ (NF-κβ) and hypoxia-inducible factor-1 alpha (HIF-1α) was positively correlated with AHI, and was significantly higher in those with severe OSA than in control and mild-moderate OSA groups. In contrast, expression of surfactant protein D protein (SPDP) was negatively correlated with AHI, and was significantly lower in those with severe OSA than in control and mild-moderate OSA groups. Therapy with CPAP lowered NF-κβ and HIF-1α, and increased SPDP protein levels.

Lu D et al. Bosn J Basic Med Sci. 2016 Oct 18.

☐

Sleep quality and physical activity improve during CPAP treatment of OSA. Physical activity and sleep quality were examined pre- and post- (3-8 months) CPAP treatment in 62 patients diagnosed with OSA in this prospective longitudinal study. Physical activity was measured using the International Physical Activity Questionnaire (IPAQ) and pedometer steps per day. Poor sleep quality and lower actual physical activity were correlated at baseline. Sleep quality and actual physical activity improved at 3 and 7 months.

Jean RE et al. J Phys Act Health. 2016 Dec 20:1-24.

☐

Treatment with CPAP reverses the impaired gait control present in some patients with OSA. In a prospective controlled study, gait performance was evaluated by stride time variability before and after 8 weeks of CPAP treatment in 12 non-obese patients with severe OSA (AHI = 46.3 ± 11.7) and 10 healthy matched subjects. At baseline, patients with OSA had higher stride time variability and step width compared to controls. Spatiotemporal gait parameters and cognition when walking improved to the levels seen in control subjects during CPAP treatment.
Baillieul S et al. Ann Phys Rehabil Med. 2016 Sep;59S:e118-e119.

☐

Good adherence to CPAP therapy for OSA enhances men's intimate relationships with their bed partners. Seventy three men with newly-diagnosed OSA were assessed before and after 1 year of CPAP treatment. Median CPAP use was 4.3 hours daily. Using CPAP improved intimate relationships directly as well as indirectly by decreasing daytime sleepiness (ESS) and increasing activity levels.
Lai AY et al. Sleep Breath. 2016 May;20(2):543-51.

☐

Prophylactic CPAP in the postoperative period following high-risk abdominal surgery reduces the incidence of pneumonia, atelectasis and pulmonary complications in patients *without* OSA. A meta-regression analysis of 11 RCTs involving adult patients (362 and 363 patients in CPAP and control groups, respectively) showed that continuous was better than intermittent CPAP in preventing pulmonary complications, but that the beneficial effect was less apparent at higher levels of CPAP.
Singh PM et al. Lung. 2016 Feb 19.

☐

Therapy with CPAP does not significantly reduce long-term adverse cardiovascular outcomes in non-sleepy patients with OSA and CAD. The RICCADSA is a single-center, prospective RCT that randomized 244 consecutive non-sleepy (ESS < 10) patients with OSA (AHI ≥ 15) and newly revascularized CAD to APAP or no PAP arms. At a median follow-up of 57 months, incidence of the primary endpoint (first event of repeat revascularization, MI, stroke or CV mortality) did not differ significantly between groups. However, on-treatment analysis demonstrated a

significant CV risk reduction in the group that used APAP for ≥ 4 hours nightly.
Peker Y et al. Am J Respir Crit Care Med. 2016 Feb 25.

☐

Continuous positive airway pressure therapy in hospitalized patients with OSA does not significantly alter hospital length of stay, readmission rate or time to readmission. Investigators conducted a retrospective review of data from 413 consecutive OSA patients using CPAP therapy who were admitted to the general medical ward. Sixty-four percent of patients received CPAP during their hospitalization, and this group were more likely to have CHF, peripheral vascular disease and uncomplicated DM compared to those who did not get CPAP therapy.
Kamel G et al. Sleep Breath. 2016 Mar 5.

☐

Continuous positive airway pressure is more effective than MADs in the treatment of OSA. A meta-analysis of 77 RCTs compared the treatment effects of conservative management, CPAP or MAD for adult patients with OSA. Both CPAP and MAD significantly improved AHI (-25.4 and -9.3, respectively) and ESS. Mean AHI and ESS scores were lower for CPAP in direct comparisons.
Sharples LD et al. Sleep Med Rev. 2016 Jun;27:108-24.

☐

Continuous positive airway pressure therapy is more effective than MADs in reducing daytime sleepiness in patients with OSA. A meta-analysis of 67 published RCTs, consisting of 6,873 patients, showed that ESS scores were reduced by 2.5 and 1.7 points by CPAP and MAD, respectively, compared to controls.
Bratton DJ et al. Lancet Respir Med. 2015 Oct 20.

☐

Continuous positive airway pressure is more effective than sleep position modification therapy in patients with supine OSA. In a meta-analysis of RCTs comparing positional modification techniques to placebo or other OSA therapies, beneficial reductions in time spent supine and in AHI were observed with sleep position therapy, but its effectiveness was inferior to that of CPAP.

Barnes H et al. Sleep Med Rev. 2016 Nov 18.

☐
Acute application of CPAP does not cause hemodynamic compromise in patients with hypertrophic cardiomyopathy. Prevalence of OSA is high in patients with hypertrophic cardiomyopathy (HCM), a disorder characterized by LV outflow tract (LVOT) obstruction, HF and sudden death. This study investigated the acute effects of CPAP on hemodynamics and cardiac performance in 26 patients with hypertrophic cardiomyopathy (12 non-obstructive and 14 obstructive HCM [LVOT gradient pressure > 30 mmHg). Beat-to-beat BP measurements and ECG were continuously monitored in wake subjects lying in a supine position. Echocardiography was performed at rest and again after 20 min of nasal CPAP (1.5 and 10 cmH2O) interposed by 10 min without CPAP. Continuous positive airway pressure at 10 cmH2O decreased right atrial size, RV relaxation, left atrial volume, and RV outflow acceleration time, but did not alter BP, cardiac output, stroke volume, HR, LVEF or LV outflow tract gradient.
Nerbass FB et al. Chest. 2016 Nov;150(5):1050-1058.

☐
Expiratory pressure relief decreases CPAP efficacy for OSA if not corrected for at the time of CPAP titration. Positive airway pressure devices (CPAP and APAP) with and without pressure relief features (PRF) were exposed to bench-simulated obstructive apneas. When PRF was activated, CPAP settings obtained without PRF were associated with lower mean pressures and more breathing events.
Zhu K et al. J Clin Sleep Med. 2015 Nov 6.

☐
Providing heated humidification via heated breathing tubes during CPAP therapy improves QOL, and decreases sleepiness and adverse effects in patients with nasopharyngeal complaints. Seventy two patients with OSA were divided based on risk of nasopharyngeal complaints, and were randomly assigned to APAP therapy with or without heated humidification for 6 weeks. There was no significant difference in treatment adherence between the heated humidification and non-heated humidification groups. In the nasopharyngeal complaint risk group, heated humidification significantly improved ESS scores,

nasopharyngeal symptoms and daily functioning (FOSQ).

Nilius G et al. Sleep Breath. 2016 Mar;20(1):43-9.

☐

Therapy using CPAP in patients with moderate-severe OSA is cost-effective. This is a retrospective, case-crossover study that compared changes in ESS, HRQOL and costs in 373 OSA patients before and after using CPAP. Improved VAS scores for EQ-5D (+ 5 points) and ESS (- 10 points) were noted. There was a significant mean gain in QALY of 0.05 per patient per year (0.07 among compliers and -0.04 in non-compliers). Incremental cost-effectiveness ratio during CPAP treatment was €51,147 and €1,544 per QALY during the first and second year, respectively.

Català R et al. Arch Bronconeumol. 2016 Sep;52(9):461-9.

☐

The AASM recommends not using ASV to treat CSA in patients with chronic HF, an LVEF of ≤ 45%, and moderate-severe CSA. This is an update of the AASM's 2012 systematic review and meta-analyses on the indications of ASV for the treatment of CSA related to CHF. This recommendation was based on an increased risk of cardiac mortality in patients with an LVEF of ≤ 45% and moderate-severe CSA-predominant SDB seen in the SERVE-HF trial. The paper provided an option level recommendation for the use of ASV in the treatment of CSA associated with HF in patients with an LVEF > 45% and mild CSA.

Aurora RN et al. J Clin Sleep Med. 2016 Apr 12.

☐

The increased risk of cardiovascular death in patients with HF (LVEF ≤ 45%) treated with ASV for CSA in the SERVE-HF trial occurred in patients not previously admitted to a hospital and in those with poor LV function. In a secondary multistate modelling analysis, investigators analyzed the associations between ASV and individual components of the primary endpoint, namely time to first event of death from any cause, life-saving CV intervention, or unplanned hospital admission for worsening HF. Use of ASV increased the risk of CV death without previous hospital admission in patients with LVEF ≤ 30%. The ASV group had increased risk of both (a) CV death without previous hospital admission and (b) CV death after a life-saving event vs. controls. The increased risk of CV death without previous hospital admission for worsening HF correlated with LVEF. Risk of hospital admission for worsening HF was associated with LVEF and CSR.

Eulenburg C et al. Lancet Respir Med. 2016 Nov;4(11):873-881.

☐

Adaptive servo ventilation has differing effects on hemodynamic parameters in patients with HF and CSR vs. healthy individuals. Hemodynamic parameters were continuously monitored for 1 hour in 27 patients with HF and CSR and 15 healthy controls at baseline, and during and after ASV intervention. Stroke volume index rose during ASV intervention in HF patients; there was also a trend towards greater parasympathetic nervous activity in this group. Stroke volume fell and

sympathetic nervous activity trended higher in normal controls. The favorable hemodynamic effects of ASV were observed in HF patients with CSR who had mitral regurgitation, increased LV filling pressures, preserved RV function, normal resting BP, and non-ischemic cause of HF.
Spießhöfer J et al. Heart Vessels. 2016 Jul;31(7):1117-30.

☐
Eighteen months of ASV therapy does not significantly impact cardiovascular death, or combined cardiovascular death and hospital readmissions, in patients with CHF and CSR. In this retrospective analysis, 75 patients with CHF (NYHA classes II-IV and LVEF ≤ 45%; receiving optimal medical therapy) and CSR (≥ 25% of sleeping time) were either treated with ASV for > 3-18 months (n = 31) or served as controls (n = 44). The two groups did not differ significantly in terms of CV death (16% [control] vs. 3% [ASV]), but there was a trend toward better CV event-free survival in the ASV group.
Hetland A et al. Scand Cardiovasc J. 2016 Dec 7:1-8.

☐
Early application of ASV in patients presenting with acute cardiogenic pulmonary edema in the emergency room decreases the need for endotracheal intubation and reduces hospital length of stay.
Consecutive patients (n = 198) were given either standard therapy (O_2 inhalation and vasodilators; n = 80) or ASV in addition to standard therapy (n = 118) in the emergency room immediately after they were diagnosed with acute cardiogenic pulmonary edema. Patients were intubated when oxygenation remained insufficient despite treatment. The ASV group had significantly lower rates of endotracheal intubation (3% vs. 21%), shorter intensive care and/or high care unit length of stay (1.9 ± 2.1 vs. 5.3 ± 6.8 days), and briefer hospitalization period (19.3 ± 11.0 vs. 26.3 ± 16.6 days) than the group that was given only standard treatment.
Kinoshita M et al. J Cardiol. 2016 Jun 29.

☐
Adaptive servo ventilation prevents cardiac death in patients with advanced HF. This report described the clinical outcomes at 2-year follow-up of 85 patients with advanced HF (71% NYHA class IV) placed on ASV irrespective of SDB. Patients who continued ASV therapy had

significantly lower all-cause mortality and cardiac death rate compared to those who discontinued therapy. Use of ASV was also associated with improvements in sympathetic activity, LVEF, NYHA class and plasma level of BNP.

Imamura T et al. Int Heart J. 2016 Jan 19;57(1):47-52.

☐
Shorter duration of HF predicts better responsiveness to ASV treatment in patients with advanced HF. Servo ventilation therapy was given to 47 patients with advanced HF (74% were NYHA class IV, and 38% were inotrope infusion-dependent). Left ventricular ejection fraction increased by ≥ 5% during the 6-month study period in 26% of patients. Shorter duration of HF (< 1,720 days) significantly predicted responsiveness to ASV therapy and was associated with improved HF symptoms, recovery of renal function, and lower readmissions compared to a longer duration of HF.

Imamura T et al. Int Heart J. 2016 Mar 22;57(2):198-203.

☐
Adaptive servo ventilation improves cardiac function, symptoms, exercise capacity and cardiac sympathetic nerve activity in persons with CHF and CSA-CSR. Nuclear imaging, exercise capacity, NYHA class and cardiac sympathetic nerve activity were evaluated in 31 subjects with CHF (LVEF ≤ 40%) and CSA-CSR who had been randomized to ASV therapy or to conservative non-ASV treatment. After 6 months, AHI, LVEF, exercise capacity, NYHA class, and cardiac sympathetic nerve activity were better in the ASV group.

Toyama T et al. J Nucl Cardiol. 2016 Jul 7.

☐
Adaptive servo ventilation improves QOL in patients with chronic HF and CSR. In a nurse-led HF clinic, 51 patients (NYHA class III-IV and/or LVEF ≤ 40%) with CSR were randomized to receive ASV or to a control arm. Quality of life was assessed at randomization and after 3 months using the Minnesota Living with Heart Failure Questionnaire. Quality of life scores improved in the ASV group in both per-protocol and intention-to-treat analyses.

Olseng MW et al. J Clin Nurs. 2016 Jun 6.

☐

Patients with CSA have better sleep quality when using ASV compared to CPAP. Twenty seven patients with SDB (AHI of 55 ± 24 and CAI of 23 ± 18 at baseline) were enrolled in a prospective, multicenter, observational trial. Following an automated ASV titration without technician intervention, 26 patients used ASV at home for 3 months. Mean adherence was 4.2 hours per night. Sleep quality was better on ASV than CPAP. Epworth Sleepiness Scale decreased significantly from 12.8 to 7.8.
Javaheri S et al. Chest. 2015 Dec 1;148(6):1454-61.

☐

Servo ventilation and auto-bilevel PAP reduces sleep disturbance in patients with sleep-onset insomnia. This is a nonrandomized controlled retrospective study in which 74 patients, predominantly psychiatric, with severe chronic sleep-onset insomnia and comorbid sleep apnea were manually titrated with ASV or auto-bilevel PAP after failing CPAP or BPAP. Psychiatric conditions included depression, anxiety, traumatic exposure, claustrophobia, panic attacks and PTSD. Patients were classified based on PAP compliance at 1-year follow-up as PAP users (> 20 hours per week) or partial PAP users (< 20 hours per week). Compared to the partial PAP user group, PAP users had significantly greater reductions in global insomnia severity and sleep-onset insomnia.
Krakow B et al. Prim Care Companion CNS Disord. 2016 Sep 29;18(5).

☐

Oronasal masks are associated with higher residual AHI and higher CPAP pressure requirements than nasal or nasal pillow masks. This is a retrospective comparison of 358 mask prescriptions (46% oronasal masks, 35% nasal masks and 19% nasal pillow masks) for CPAP therapy of sleep apnea. Baseline AHI, BMI, and waist or neck circumference were similar for all mask types. Levels of CPAP were higher for oronasal masks than nasal pillow or nasal masks (median [interquartile range] of 12 [10-15.5], 11 [8-12.5] and 10 [8-12] cmH_2O, respectively). Residual AHI was also higher for oronasal masks than nasal pillow and nasal masks (median of 11.3, 6.7 and 6.4 events per hour, respectively). Higher CPAP requirements were independently predicted by oronasal mask type, age, AHI and BMI.
Deshpande S et al. J Clin Sleep Med. 2016 Sep 15;12(9):1263-8.

☐

Oronasal masks for CPAP therapy increase obstructive events in patients with OSA. Eighteen patients underwent PSG during midazolam-induced sleep. Nasoendoscopy was used to continuously visualize the retroglossal area. During CPAP titration, flow was changed from nasal to oronasal or oral routes. Oronasal and oral masks promoted obstructive events in 66% and 87% of patients, respectively. Stable breathing was observed endoscopically with the nasal route, whereas there were reductions in the distance between the epiglottis and the tongue base with the oronasal route, and in the retroglossal space with the oral route.
Andrade RG et al. Chest. 2016 Dec;150(6):1194-1201.

☐

Unintentional leaks are greater when oronasal masks are used during CPAP therapy. In this systematic review, factors associated with greater unintentional leak were oronasal mask, presence of nasal obstruction, male gender, older age, higher BMI and central fat distribution.
Lebret M et al. Chest. 2016 Dec 13.

☐

Persistent mouth opening during CPAP therapy for OSA is more common among users of oronasal masks compared to nasal masks.

Mouth opening was recorded during a type 4 sleep study in 38 patients with OSA. Compared to nasal mask users, patients using oronasal masks had more nasal obstruction, greater mouth opening and higher ODIs. Male gender and nasal obstruction contributed to mouth opening.

Lebret M et al. Respirology. 2015 Oct;20(7):1123-30.

☐

Mandibular advancement devices improve UA collapsibility in patients with OSA, especially in those with lower loop gain and mild anatomic derangement. Investigators of this randomized crossover study evaluated how MADs modify four OSA phenotypic traits, namely UA anatomy, UA muscle function, arousal threshold and loop gain. Sleep studies performed on 14 OSA patients with and without using their MADs showed that the latter significantly lowered AHIs and improved UA anatomy and collapsibility. In multivariate analysis, both baseline passive UA collapsibility and loop gain were independent predictors of AHI reduction.

Edwards BA et al. Am J Respir Crit Care Med. 2016 Dec 1;194(11):1413-1422.

☐

Most patients with moderate-severe OSA, who are non-complaint to CPAP therapy, can be successfully treated using oral appliances. Overall success rate of custom-made MADs was 75% in a retrospective study of 106 OSA patients who were non-adherent to CPAP treatment. A ≤ 50% reduction in baseline AHI during a nocturnal respiratory polygraphy at follow-up was considered as a therapeutic failure. The average time for follow-up was 12 months.

Gjerde K et al. J Oral Rehabil. 2016 Apr;43(4):249-58.

☐

It is cost-effective to treat OSA patients who have a high cardiovascular risk with CPAP and to treat patients with mild-moderate OSA and low cardiovascular risk with dental devices. A study funded by the French National Authority for Health reported that CPAP was associated with a gain of 0.62 QALY vs. no treatment, resulting in an ICER of 10,128 EUR/QALY for patients with a high CV risk. In contrast, ICER of dental devices vs. no treatment varied between 32,976 - 45,579 EUR/QALY (for moderate and mild OSA, respectively), and ICER of CPAP vs. dental devices was over 256,000 EUR/QALY for those with low CV risk.

Poullié AI et al. Int J Technol Assess Health Care. 2016 Mar 9:1-9.

☐
Many older adults perceive MADs as being ineffective. Surveys were mailed to adults aged ≥ 65 years who were prescribed MAD therapy for OSA. Of the 39 respondents (response rate of 30%), only 36% described that regular MAD use was effective in managing their OSA, 39% felt confident about using MADs regularly, 41% stated that people in their life supported their therapy, and 38% noted that health care staff would help them use their devices.
Carballo NJ et al. Clin Ther. 2016 Oct 14.

☐
Better treatment response to OSA can be expected for custom-made MADs than ready-made MADs. Twenty five patients with mild OSA and daytime sleepiness were entered into this randomized crossover trial comparing the effectiveness of custom-made vs. ready-made MADs in treating OSA. Each intervention was given for 3 months, with a washout period of 2 weeks before crossover. Complete treatment response was significantly higher for custom-made MADs than ready-made MADs (64% and 24%, respectively). Treatment failures were also significantly different at 4% (custom-made MAD) vs. 36%. Excessive sleepiness (ESS ≥10) persisted in 33% and 66% of custom-made MAD and ready-made MAD groups, respectively. Quality of life scales improved only in subjects who used custom-made MADs.
Johal A et al. J Clin Sleep Med. 2016 Oct 20.

☐
Increasing the degree of mandibular advancement using oral devices does not always result in improvements in AHI. This systematic review of 13 RCTs investigated the efficacy of MADs in reducing AHI in subjects with OSA. Analysis revealed that advancements greater than 50% did not significantly increase success rate.
Bartolucci ML et al. Sleep Breath. 2016 Jan 15.

☐
Sleep studies using remotely controlled mandibular protrusion technology accurately predicts MAD treatment outcomes. This study validated a remotely controlled mandibular protrusion device method during PSG in 42 subjects with OSA (AHI > 10) before starting MAD treatment. A prediction of "success" or "failure" of treatment was made

for each subject based on a rule of ≤ 1 respiratory event per 5 minutes of supine REM sleep. Polysomnography was used to verify response to MAD therapy (i.e., treatment AHI < 10 with 50% reduction). Baseline AHI was 31.5 ± 20.5, and 39% of subjects had severe OSA (AHI > 30). This method had a sensitivity of 81.8%, specificity of 92.9%, PPV of 90% and NPV of 86.7% in predicting outcomes.
Sutherland K et al. J Clin Sleep Med. 2016 Nov 28.

☐
Determining the optimal protrusion position using a remote-controlled mandibular positioner titration system predicts effectiveness of MAD therapy. Four articles and 5 conference abstracts, consisting of 254 patients with OSA, were included in this systematic review. Predicted mean AHI between the remote-controlled mandibular positioner and treatment outcomes from MAD were significantly correlated.
Kastoer C et al. J Clin Sleep Med. 2016 Oct 15;12(10):1411-1421.

☐
Early control of OSA by MAD is a marker of long-term adherence. Long-term adherence to MADs was prospectively evaluated in 279 patients who were followed for a median of 1,002 days. Sixty-three percent of patients continued to use MADs and, in adjusted multivariate analysis, significant predictors of adherence included an early ≥ 50% reduction in AHI and early complete resolution of symptoms. Treatment inefficacy, discomfort and adverse effects were the main reasons given for discontinuation of treatment.
Attali V et al. Sleep Med. 2016 Nov - Dec;27-28:107-114.

☐

Upper airway surgery for OSA decreases AHI, improves CPAP adherence and reduces required CPAP pressure. Eleven articles, which involved 323 patients, were included in this meta-analysis. Upper airway surgery reduced CPAP by a mean of 1.40 cmH_2O and increased in adherence by 0.62-hours.

Ayers CM et al. ORL J Otorhinolaryngol Relat Spec 2016 Apr 7;78(3):119-125.

☐

Upper airway surgery for OSA improves QOL – this improvement was equivalent to that seen with compliant CPAP use. A retrospective cohort study was conducted on consecutive patients receiving therapy for OSA (n = 83 [CPAP]; 83 [UA surgery]; and 79 [MAD]. Glasgow Benefit Inventory, Snoring Severity Scale, ESS and adverse effects were recorded after starting therapy (mean 34.5 months). Quality of life following UA surgery significantly improved vs. complaint MAD and noncompliant CPAP groups. Improvement in the Snoring Severity Scale was similar for CPAP and UA surgery, and both were superior to MAD.

Woods CM et al. Clin Otolaryngol. 2016 Dec;41(6):762-770.

☐

Tonsillectomy can effectively treat adult patients with mild-moderate OSA (AHI < 30) who have large tonsils. A meta-analysis of 17 studies (n = 216 patients) showed a reduction in AHI by 65.2% (from 40.5 ± 28.9 to 14.1 ± 17.1 in 203 patients), an improvement in SaO_2min (from 77.7 ± 11.9% to 85.5 ± 8.2% in 186 patients), and a decrease in ESS (from 11.6 ± 3.7 to 6.1 ± 3.9 in 125 patients). Tonsillectomy resulted in an 85.2% success rate (i.e., AHI < 20 and ≥ 50% reduction) and a 57.4% cure rate in 54 patients. A preoperative AHI < 30 was a significant predictor of surgical success and cure. Tonsillectomy success rate, cure rate and mean postoperative AHI were 100%, 84% and 2.4 ± 2.1 per hour among patients with a preoperative AHI < 30; and 72.4%, 34.4% and 14.3 ± 13.9 per hour for the group with a preoperative AHI ≥ 30.

Camacho M et al. Laryngoscope. 2016 Sep;126(9):2176-86.

☐

A single night of transcutaneous electrical stimulation of the pharyngeal dilator muscles improves UA obstruction in patients with OSA. In a randomized sham-controlled trial, 36 patients with OSA were assigned to one night of transcutaneous electrical stimulation of the UA dilator muscles and one night of sham stimulation. Response, defined as > 25% reduction in 4% ODI compared with sham stimulation and/or 4%ODI < 5 in the active treatment night, improved significantly during active treatment. A 47.2% positive response rate was observed in patients with mild-moderate OSA; and ODI and AHI were significantly reduced by 10.0 and 9.1, respectively. Stimulation was well tolerated
Pengo MF et al. Thorax. 2016 Oct;71(10):923-31.

☐

Rapid maxillary expansion significantly reduces AHI in children with OSA. In a meta-analysis, which included 10 articles (n = 215 children with OSA), mean AHI was reduced by -6.86 following rapid maxillary expansion.
Machado-Júnior AJ et al. Med Oral Patol Oral Cir Bucal. 2016 Jul 1;21(4):e465-9.

☐

Weight reduction through a lifestyle modification program reduces OSA severity and daytime sleepiness. In this RCT, a dietician-led lifestyle modification was more effective than usual care in reducing AHI, BMI and ESS at 4 and 12 months in 104 patients with moderate-severe OSA.
Ng SS et al. Chest. 2015 Nov 1;148(5):1193-203.

☐

Moderate energy restricted diet reduces disease severity in obese persons with OSA. Twenty one obese adults with OSA (AHI ≥ 5) were included in this 16-week RCT. Subjects who followed an energy-restricted diet (-3347·2 kJ/d [-800 kcal/d]) had significantly greater reductions in weight, AHI and plasma adrenaline levels (sympathetic activity), and higher SaO_2min, compared to those who did not alter their food intake.
Fernandes JF et al. Br J Nutr. 2015 Dec;114(12):2022-31.

☐

A person's weight influences the effectiveness of positional therapy to treat snoring in patients with OSA. Investigators assessed subjective snoring severity with a visual analogue scale and objective snoring index (number of snoring events per hour) using acoustic analysis in 25 adults with positional OSA who were using a head-positioning pillow. Both measures improved significantly in normal-weight patients, whereas only subjective snoring intensity decreased in patients who were overweight.
Chen WC et al. Sci Rep. 2015 Dec 11;5:18188.

☐

A semi-recumbent sleep position significantly decreases the severity of OSA in patients with HF. Polysomnograpy was performed on 30 patients with OSA and HF while they slept in a semi-recumbent (45-degree elevated) or supine position. Mean AHIs were 17.8 ± 12.1 and 30.8 ± 20.7 while lying in semi-recumbent or supine positions, respectively. Percentage of sleep time with SaO_2 < 90%, SaO_2min and ODI were also better in the semi-recumbent sleep position.
Basoglu OK et al. J Card Fail. 2015 Oct;21(10):842-7.

☐

A lateral sleep position has beneficial effects on SDB in patients with HF. Persons with moderate-severe, but stable, HF and SDB (AHI ≥ 15) were included in this study. Twenty nine and 91 patients had predominant OSA and CSA, respectively. Positional sleep apnea was noted in 76% of OSA patients and 53% of CSA patients. In both groups, a change from a supine to lateral sleep position markedly decreased AHI. Patients with OSA had greater improvement in disease severity than those with CSA.
Pinna GD et al. Eur J Heart Fail. 2015 Dec;17(12):1302-9.

☐

Exercise therapy, as a sole intervention, improves clinical outcomes in adult patients with OSA. Eight articles, consisting of 182 participants, were included in this meta-analysis. Using a random effects model, exercise was associated with decreased AHI, reduced ESS and lower BMI.
Aiello KD et al. Respir Med. 2016 Jul;116:85-92.

☐

Moderate-to-vigorous physical activity lowers the risk of OSA. These are the results from a multicenter population-based study, the Hispanic Community Health Study/Study of Latinos (n = 14,087 participants aged 18-74 years). Compared to inactivity, moderate-vigorous physical activity lowered the odds of mild OSA (AHI ≥ 5) and moderate-severe OSA (AHI ≥ 15). Medium-high levels of transportation activity and moderate-vigorous recreational physical activity lowered the odds of mild OSA and both mild and moderate-severe OSA, respectively. There was no significant correlation between vigorous physical activity and OSA.
Murillo R et al. Prev Med. 2016 Dec;93:183-188.

☐

Aerobic exercise training, by decreasing overnight fluid shift and enlarging the cross-sectional area of the UA, reduces sleep apnea severity. In this randomized trial, patients with SDB (OSA or CSA [AHI > 15]) and CAD were assigned to 4 weeks of exercise training (n = 17) or control (n = 17). Each subject underwent PSG, and measurements of fluid volumes (leg, thorax and neck) and UA cross-sectional area before and after sleep, at baseline and during follow-up. Compared to controls, the exercise group had significantly lower AHI, less overnight change in leg

fluid volume, and greater overnight change in UA cross-sectional area.
Mendelson M et al. Eur Respir J. 2016 Jul;48(1):142-50.

☐

Structured physical exercise lowers the odds for OSA. A total of 5,453 individuals underwent PSG, answered the International Physical Activity Questionnaire, and were classified as "exercisers" or "non-exercisers" (56%) and as "occupationally active" or "occupationally non-active" (75%). Apnea hypopnea indices were significantly higher in non-exercisers vs. exercisers as well as, surprisingly, in active vs. non-active occupations. In addition, SaO_2min was lower and time with $SaO_2 < 90\%$ was longer among non-exercisers. In multinomial logistic regression, structured exercise was shown to significantly lower the likelihood of developing moderate and severe OSA. Occupational activity did not replace the benefits of regular exercise.
da Silva RP et al. J Clin Sleep Med. 2016 Oct 20.

☐

Combination therapy using supplemental O_2 and a hypnotic agent improves OSA in patients with mild-moderately collapsible upper airways. This regimen lowered loop gain and raised the arousal threshold. Twenty patients with OSA received combination therapy (3 mg eszopiclone and 40% O_2) versus control (placebo and sham air) with 1 week between arms in this single-blinded randomized crossover study. Clinical and research PSGs were conducted in each study condition. Compared to controls, combination therapy significantly reduced AHI (51.9 ± 6.2 vs. 29.5 ± 5.3), decreased ventilation associated with arousal and and lowered loop gain. Subjects who responded to combination therapy (i.e., reduction in AHI by > 50% to below 15) had less severe OSA, less UA collapsibility and greater UA muscle responsiveness.
Edwards BA et al. Sleep. 2016 Nov 1;39(11):1973-1983.

☐

Oral carbocysteine, an antioxidant, reduces oxidative stress in patients with moderate-severe OSA. In this clinical trial, 40 patients with OSA were randomized to receive either nighttime CPAP or carbocysteine (1,500 mg daily). Questionnaires, biochemical analyses and PSGs were completed before and after 6 weeks of treatment. In addition, subjects in the carbocysteine group underwent ultrasonography to assess endothelial function. Compliance was higher in the carbocysteine group compared to the CPAP group. Subjects in both groups had significant improvements in AHI, snoring volume, ESS, 90% O_2 desaturation, SaO_2min and levels of plasma malondialdehyde, superoxide dismutase and nitric oxide compared to baseline. Mean SaO_2, ODI and endothelin-1 level improved in the CPAP group but not in the carbocysteine group. Finally, ultrasonography in the carbocysteine group demonstrated reductions in the intima-media thickness but no significant change in flow-mediated dilation.

Wu K et al. PLoS One. 2016 Feb 5;11(2):e0148519.

☐
Spironolactone reduces BP and decreases OSA severity in patients with resistant HTN and moderate-severe OSA. Thirty patients with resistant HTN and OSA (AHI > 15) were randomly assigned to spironolactone (in addition to their original antihypertensive medication) or control, and were followed for 12 weeks. Compared to control, therapy significantly reduced AHI, hypopnea index, ODI, clinical and ambulatory BP, and plasma aldosterone level. No side effects were reported by the study participants.

Yang L et al. Clin Exp Hypertens. 2016 Jul 1:1-5.

☐
Success rate of oral pressure therapy for OSA varies between 25% and 37%. Treatment success was defined as ≥ 50% reduction from baseline AHI and residual AHI ≤ 10. Response was better in patients with retropalatal collapse, but efficacy did not correlate with disease severity.

Nigam G et al. Sleep Breath. 2015 Oct 19.

☐
Nasopharyngeal stenting is less effective in improving AHI in patients with OSA compared to CPAP. First-night treatment success was determined for nasopharyngeal stenting and CPAP titration in 8 patients with untreated OSA. Mean AHIs were 31 (pretreatment), 19 (stent) and 8 (CPAP). Responder rate for nasopharyngeal stents was 50%, and no complications were reported.

Traxdorf M et al. Eur Arch Otorhinolaryngol. 2015 Nov 2.

☐

Long-term nocturnal O$_2$ therapy improves SDB, cardiac function and QOL in patients with chronic HF and CSA. A post hoc analysis of 2 trials of 97 patients with chronic HF and CSA who received 12 weeks of LTOT or no LTOT showed that O$_2$ therapy was associated with greater improvements in AHI, LVEF, NYHA functional class and Specific Activity Scale. The frequency of premature ventricle beats was not reduced by LTOT except in the subgroup with NYHA class > III and AHI > 20.
Nakao YM et al. Heart Vessels. 2016 Feb;31(2):165-72.

☐

Cardiac resynchronization therapy reduces apneic events in patients with CSA. Twenty two trials were included in this systematic review of the effects of cardiac pacing on SDB in patients with or without HF. Unlike cardiac resynchronization therapy, atrial overdrive pacing did not decrease apneic events in those with CSA.
Anastasopoulos DL et al. Heart Fail Rev. 2016 Sep;21(5):579-90.

☐

Oropharyngeal exercise therapy reduces the severity of mild-moderate OSA and increases CPAP compliance. Twenty patients with mild-moderate OSA performed oropharyngeal exercise therapy to increase pharyngeal muscle tone for 3 months. Soft palate, tongue, and facial muscle exercises were repeated 10 times at 5 sets each day. Polysomnography was performed at baseline and repeated at the end of the study. Unlike BMI, which did not change significantly, there was a significant reduction in neck circumference. Improvements were also observed in snoring intensity, daytime sleepiness, witnessed apneas, SE, N3 sleep, SaO$_2$min, duration of SaO$_2$ < 90%, and arousal index.
Verma RK et al. Sleep Breath. 2016 Mar 18.

☐

Inspiratory muscle strength training improves sleep, arousals, BP and plasma catecholamine levels in patients with OSA who are unable to use CPAP therapy. This study enrolled 24 adults with OSA who were randomized to placebo or inspiratory muscle strength training (performed 5 minutes each day for 6 weeks). Polysomnography was performed at the start and at the end of the study. Inspiratory muscle strength training reduced systolic and diastolic BP, plasma norepinephrine levels and nighttime arousals as well as improved sleep (PSQI), but did not change AHI, compared to placebo.

Vranish JR et al. Sleep. 2016 Jun 1;39(6):1179-85.

☐

Adherence to CPAP therapy has remained persistently low over the past 20 years. A systematic literature review of 82 papers published from 1994-2015 revealed an overall CPAP non-adherence rate of 34.1% based on a 7-hour per night sleep time. There was no significant improvement in CPAP adherence noted over the 20-year time period, and behavioral interventions improved adherence rates by only an average of ~1 h per night.
Rotenberg BW et al. J Otolaryngol Head Neck Surg. 2016 Aug 19;45(1):43.

☐

Many factors influence adherence to CPAP therapy of OSA in clinical studies. Data from the Apnea Positive Pressure Long-term Efficacy Study (APPLES) cohort suggest that randomization to active therapy, belief that one is receiving active (vs. sham) treatment, older age, and presence of CV disorders positively affected CPAP adherence, whereas nasal congestion and anxiety had negative effects.
Budhiraja R et al. J Clin Sleep Med. 2015 Oct 22.

☐

Composite indices of sleep apnea severity are better at predicting CPAP adherence and subjective treatment outcomes than baseline AHI or ESS. Researchers performed PSG on 323 patients. Indices (e.g., Sleep Apnea Severity Index, and Modified Sleep Apnea Severity Index) and, to a lesser degree, baseline AHI, but not baseline ESS, predicted adherence to CPAP therapy at 6 months. However, only the composite metrics predicted changes in Sleep Apnea Quality of Life Index.
Balakrishnan K et al. J Clin Sleep Med. 2016 Feb 1.

☐

Non-obese patients are less adherent with CPAP therapy. Sleep and anthropometric data were obtained at baseline and during follow-up (up to 22 months) in 163 patients with OSA (AHI > 5). Fifty-four percent of patients were non-obese (BMI < 30). Compared to the obese group, non-obese patients were more likely to report non-use of CPAP at follow-up (13% vs. 36% [non-obese]), have lower objective CPAP compliance (6.4 ± 0.4 vs. 5.1 ± 0.4 hours per night [non-obese]), and have a higher

proportion of low respiratory arousal threshold (60% vs. 86% [non-obese]).
Gray EL et al. J Clin Sleep Med. 2016 Sep 13.

☐

Initial and late insomnia reduces adherence to PAP therapy in non-obese patients with OSA. A prospective study of PAP adherence was conducted in 798 subjects with moderate-severe OSA (AHI ≥ 15) in the Icelandic Sleep Apnea Cohort. The PAP devices were returned within the first year in 15.5% of patients and another 21.4% were returned later. At long-term follow-up (6.7 ± 1.2 years), 63.2% of patients were still on PAP therapy. Patients who quit therapy within the first year had more baseline symptoms of initial and late insomnia than long-term PAP users. After adjustments, initial and late insomnia were significantly associated with early quitting in subjects with BMI < 30 but not in those with BMI ≥ 30.
Eysteinsdottir B et al. J Sleep Res. 2016 Dec 15.

☐

Neighborhood income level of sleepy patients with severe OSA influences their acceptance/purchase of CPAP devices in a co-payment healthcare system. Overall CPAP acceptance rate was low in this study. Residence in a higher-income neighborhood was associated with better CPAP acceptance compared to living in a low-income area, with a cumulative incidence at 6 months of 52% and 43%, respectively.
Kendzerska T et al. Ann Am Thorac Soc. 2015 Oct 16.

☐

Adherence to PAP treatment among children is low but is better if a family member is also on PAP therapy. A retrospective chart review identified 56 children (< 18 years of age) with a new diagnosis of OSA, and monitored objective PAP adherence at 1 week, 1 month and 3 months. Coexisting developmental disabilities were present in 32% of the children. At 3 months, overall PAP adherence was 2.8 ± 2.4 hours per night. Thirty-three percent of the children had a family member using PAP, and this group had a significantly higher average nightly PAP use.
Puri P et al. J Clin Sleep Med. 2016 Jul 15;12(7):959-63.

☐

Patterns of early PAP use impacts long-term adherence to therapy among commercial motor vehicle drivers. A retrospective chart review was conducted on 120 drivers being evaluated for OSA, of whom 53 were started on PAP therapy. Early PAP usage best predicted one-year adherence. Overall, adherence to therapy was 68.0% and 39.6% at 1 week and 1 year, respectively. Adherence at 1 year was 52.8% in the group that was adherent at week 1 compared to only 11.7% among those who were non-adherent at week 1.

Colvin LJ et al. J Clin Sleep Med. 2016 Apr 15.

☐

Persistence of UA symptoms during CPAP initiation, but not severity of UA symptoms prior to starting CPAP, predicts therapy adherence at one year. Researchers assessed the impact of UA symptoms on 1-year adherence in 536 subjects with OSA. Significant reductions in rhinorrhea, nasal stuffiness and mouth dryness occurred in subjects who continued to use CPAP compared to those who quit CPAP.

Kreivi HR et al. Respir Care. 2016 Jan 5.

☐

Heated humidification improves CPAP adherence and QOL in patients with moderate-severe OSA and nasopharyngeal symptoms. In this prospective randomized crossover study, these improvements were observed in patients residing in a tropical climate area with a high humidity level. Twenty subjects with moderate-severe OSA and complaining of nasopharyngeal symptoms were randomly assigned to 4 weeks of CPAP with or without heated humidification and then crossed over. The addition of heated humidification improved CPAP adherence on the days of use compared with conventional CPAP (5.5 ± 1.5 vs. 5.2 ± 1.4 hours per night, respectively), but did not significantly improve average hours of use for all days (4.6 ± 1.7 vs. 4.0 ± 1.7 hours per night, respectively). The heated humidification group reported better QOL (FOSQ) and had less dry/sore throat symptoms (modified XERO questionnaire).

Soudorn C et al. Respir Care. 2016 Sep;61(9):1151-9.

☐

Heated humidification improves CPAP acceptance and reduces UA

symptoms related to CPAP titration during sleep in cool environments.
Forty patients with newly diagnosed OSA were randomly assigned to receive heated humidification or non-heated humidification during CPAP titration in a cool sleeping environment. Use of a heated humidifier significantly decreased UA symptoms, improved satisfaction with initial CPAP therapy and enhanced willingness to continue CPAP use. The two groups did not differ significantly in AHI reduction, optimal CPAP setting or leak.

Li Y et al. Sleep Breath. 2016 Dec;20(4):1255-1261.

☐

Heated breathing tube humidification does not increase treatment adherence, reduce adverse effects nor improve QOL compared to conventional heated humidification in OSA patients using CPAP.
Investigators randomized 88 CPAP users to a heated humidifier plus integrated heated breathing tube or to a conventional heated humidifier for 12 months. Improvements in sleep quality and respiratory disturbance were similar in the two groups as were overall satisfaction, rate of side effects and QOL. There was no statistically significant difference in duration of nightly CPAP use.

Galetke W et al. Respiration. 2016;91(1):18-25.

☐

Choosing the right CPAP mask at initiation of therapy is important to ensure acceptance by SDB patients. Switching CPAP masks increased the likelihood of giving up PAP therapy. Initial mask acceptance rate was 81%. Out of 2,768 patients, 267 patients had 343 cases of mask switching, defined in this prospective study as replacing a mask that was used for ≥ 1 day with another type of mask. Mask switching was more frequent in women and in new PAP users. Factors that led to mask switching were poorly fitting or uncomfortable mask (39%), leaks (30%) and nasal stuffiness (6%). The likelihood of giving up PAP therapy was 7.2 times higher among mask switchers than in the group that did not switch masks.

Bachour A et al. Sleep Breath. 2016 May;20(2):733-8.

☐

Clinical monitoring by a specialist enhances adherence to CPAP therapy.
Factors affecting CPAP compliance were assessed in 138 patients with

OSA. Good compliance (CPAP ≥ 4 hours per night) was noted in 55.8% of patients, and poor compliance (< 4 hours per night) in 44.2%. Regular monitoring improved compliance with CPAP therapy.
Pelosi LB et al. Braz J Otorhinolaryngol. 2016 Jul 14.

☐
A mobile, web-based system that allows self-monitoring of PAP use, and provides real-time education and feedback improves PAP adherence. When combined with a clinic CPAP support program, this mobile system resulted in an 18% increase in nights > 4 hour of use in 30 subjects initiating PAP treatment compared to 31 controls. Percentage of nights with any use and > 4 hours of PAP use were both significantly higher in the mobile system group compared to controls at 11 weeks. The mobile system correlated significantly with percentage of nights with > 4 hours of PAP use in multivariate linear regression analysis.
Hostler JM et al. J Sleep Res. 2016 Dec 8.

☐
A CPAP adherence program using web-based telehealth reduces coaching labor compared to standard care. Authors of this non-blinded, multicenter, prospective study reported that effectiveness (CPAP efficacy and change in ESS) and adherence (daily CPAP use) of telehealth were comparable to standard CPAP education and set-up in 122 subjects with newly diagnosed OSA. Telehealth consisted of automated text messages or emails that were generated by preset parameters. Standard care involved scheduled calls on days 1, 7, 14 and 30.
Munafo D et al. Sleep Breath. 2016 Jan 11.

☐
Telemetry-triggered interventions increase early adherence to CPAP therapy. Subjects were assigned to telemetry supervision and targeted telephone support (n = 113) or control (n = 110) in the first 30 days of CPAP use. The telemetry group had higher CPAP adherence compared to the control group (5.3 hours per night on 28 of 30 nights vs. 4.6 hours per night on 27 of 30 nights, respectively).
Frasnelli M et al. J Telemed Telecare. 2016 Jun;22(4):209-14.

☐
Myofunctional therapy improves CPAP adherence in OSA patients.
Myofunctional evaluation, ESS and PSGs were evaluated in 100 men with OSA (AHI of 30.9 ± 20.6) before intervention (myofunctional therapy; CPAP; combined CPAP-myofunctional therapy; or placebo), after 3 months of intervention, and after 3 weeks of washout. Improvements in ESS, snoring and AHI were noted during active treatments, with AHI reduction being greater in the CPAP group. Improvements in ESS and snoring were maintained during the washout period in the myofunctional therapy group. Adherence to CPAP was greater in the combined CPAP-myofunctional therapy group compared to the CPAP group. Tongue and soft palate muscle strength improved in those who received myofunctional therapy.

Diaféria G et al. Sleep Breath. 2016 Dec 2.

☐

Prevalence of CSA increases in patients with acute decompensated HF and decreases during cardiac recompensation. One hundred and five patients with acute decompensated HF (NYHA class 3.2 ± 0.6, LVEF 38.5 ± 13.3%, and BNP 1299 ± 1290 pg/ml) underwent cardiorespiratory polygraphy at the time of hospital admission and again during cardiac recompensation. Prevalence of CSA at hospital admission was 77% (21% mild, 39% moderate and 40% severe based on AHI). Central hypopnea index, time spent with CSR and oxygenation improved significantly during treatment of HF; however, there were no significant changes in AHI or CSR cycle length.
Basic K et al. Sleep Med. 2016 Nov - Dec;27-28:15-19.

☐

Heart failure patients with CSA/CSR have more impaired functional state, cardiovascular anatomy and hemodynamics. Cardiovascular structure and hemodynamics were evaluated in 161 stable HF patients with LVEF ≤ 45% (mean LVEF 32.8%) and NYHA class I-III. Fifty one patients had moderate-severe CSA/CSR and 110 had no-mild CSA/CSR. Patients with CSA/CSR had more advanced NYHA class; more frequent permanent AF; lower LVEF, stroke index and cardiac index; and higher LV and RV end-diastolic diameter, ratio of early transmitral flow velocity to early diastolic septal mitral annulus velocity (E/e'), HR and systemic vascular resistance index. Significant predictors of CSA/CSR included NYHA class (the only independent predictor), AF, RV enlargement, LVEF < 35%, E/e' and stroke index < 35 ml/m^2.
Kazimierczak A et al. Med Sci Monit. 2016 Aug 25;22:2989-98.

☐

The possibility of a new-onset coronary heart disease event is significantly higher among hemodialysis patients with CSA than in those without CSA. This risk was independent of obstructive AHI. Equally important, the prevalence of CSA, but not obstructive AHI, was significantly higher in hemodialysis patients compared to non-hemodialysis patients. Hemodialysis (n = 73) and non-hemodialysis (n = 444) patients underwent PSG in order to identify OSA and CSA, and were followed for the development of new coronary heart disease events.

Both CSA prevalence and central AHI were significantly higher in the hemodialysis group, and CSA prevalence was a risk factor for new-onset coronary heart disease events independent of OSA.
Sakura M et al. Am J Nephrol. 2016;44(5):388-395.

☐

Central sleep apnea is associated with worse prognosis and longer length of stay in the coronary care unit in patients suffering from acute coronary syndrome. Respiratory polygraphy was performed during the first 24 to 72 hours of hospital admission for acute coronary syndrome. Central sleep apnea was defined as AHI >15; > 50% being central apneas. The study included 68 patients with CSA (AHI 31 ± 18) and 92 controls (AHI 7 ± 5). After adjusting for age, BMI, HTN and smoking status, CSA was related to significantly worse Killip class and more days spent in the coronary unit compared with controls. Ejection fraction did not differ between groups.
Florés M et al. PLoS One. 2016 Nov 23;11(11):e0167031.

☐

Chronic kidney disease is independently associated with CSA.
Researchers conducted a systematic review of 8 articles consisting of 313 adult patients with CKD, including 30 patients with CSA. The prevalence of CSA in CKD was 9.6%.
Nigam G et al. Sleep Breath. 2016 Sep;20(3):957-64.

☐

Central sleep apnea increases the risk of all-cause mortality in persons with non-dialyzed CKD. Researchers assessed the effect of sleep apnea on mortality risk in 1,454 subjects undergoing PSG, 7.08% of whom had CKD. There were significant associations between CKD and both severe SDB and CSA. Central sleep apnea was an independent risk factor for dying from all causes in the CKD group.
Xu J et al. Sleep Med. 2016 Nov - Dec;27-28:32-38.

☐

Transvenous diaphragmatic neurostimulation reduces the severity of CSA. An implantable device that stimulates a nerve producing diaphragmatic contractions was tested in a prospective, randomized controlled trial. A total of 151 patients with AHI ≥ 20 were assigned to stimulation (treatment; n=73) or no stimulation (control; n=78) groups. In an intention-to-treat analysis, an AHI reduction of ≥ 50% from baseline at 6 months was significantly more common in the treatment vs. control arm (51% vs. 11%). Serious adverse effects were reported in 8% and 9% of patients in the treatment and control groups, respectively. Non-serious therapy-related discomfort occurred in 37% of treated patients – all but 1% resolved after a system reprogramming.

Costanzo MR et al. Lancet. 2016 Sep 3;388(10048):974-82.

☐
Unilateral transvenous phrenic nerve stimulation improves sleep parameters, sleep symptoms and QOL in patients with CSA over 12 months of follow-up. This is a prospective, multicenter, non-randomized study of unilateral transvenous phrenic nerve stimulation in 47 patients with CSA. Polysomnography was used to evaluate SDB parameters at 3, 6 and 12-months; 41 patients completed all follow-up PSGs. There were sustained improvements in AHI (49.9 ± 15.1 vs. 27.5 ± 18.3), CAI (28.2 ± 15.0 vs. 6.0 ± 9.2), ODI (46.1 ± 19.1 vs. 26.9 ± 18.0), SE, REM sleep, sleepiness and QOL at 12 months compared with baseline. Three deaths unrelated to therapy and 5 serious adverse events occurred during the 12-month follow-up period.

Jagielski D et al. Eur J Heart Fail. 2016 Nov;18(11):1386-1393.

☐
Prevalence of OHS is higher in women, especially during post-menopause, than in men. In this prospective cohort study, PSG confirmed the diagnosis of OSA in nearly 86% of patients with a clinical suspicion of OSA, and 8% had comorbid OHS. Prevalence of OHS was significantly greater among women than in men (15.6% vs. 4.5%), and was higher in post-menopausal than pre-menopausal women (21% vs. 5.3%). Compared to men with OHS, women with OHS were significantly older, and had more HTN, DM and hypothyroidism. Independent predictors of OHS included HCO_3 and duration of $SaO_2 < 90\%$.
BaHammam AS et al. J Sleep Res. 2016 Mar 18.

☐
Obstructive sleep apnea protects against CV morbidity in patients with OHS. Researchers conducted a cross-sectional analysis of 302 patients with OHS and observed that the prevalence of CV morbidity fell significantly with increasing ODI, and the reduction was especially evident in the highest ODI tertile.
Masa JF et al. Chest. 2016 Feb 25.

☐
Bilevel positive airway pressure and CPAP therapies for severe OHS result in similar improvements in ventilatory failure, HRQOL and treatment adherence. Bilevel positive airway pressure was compared to CPAP as initial treatment for severe OHS in 60 patients in this multicenter, parallel, double blind trial. Patients were followed for 3 months, and 57 patients (BMI 55, $PaCO_2$ 60 mmHg), who completed follow-up, were included in the analysis. Treatment failure, including hospital admission, persistent ventilatory failure or non-adherence, was not different between the 2 groups (14.8% for BPAP and 13.3% for CPAP). Three-month treatment adherence (5.3 vs. 5.0 hours per night) and wake $PaCO_2$ (44.2 vs. 45.9 mmHg) were similar for BPAP and CPAP therapies as were improvements in ESS and HRQOL (SF36). The only significant predictor of persistent ventilatory failure at 3 months was baseline level of $PaCO_2$.
Howard ME et al. Thorax. 2016 Nov 15.

☐

Noninvasive ventilation is more effective in improving daytime $PaCO_2$, sleepiness and PSG parameters than lifestyle modification in OHS patients without severe OSA. Eighty six patients without severe OSA were randomized to either NIV or lifestyle modification (control) and were followed for 2 months. Compared to lifestyle modification, NIV resulted in significantly greater improvements in $PaCO_2$ (-6 vs. -2.8 mmHg), serum bicarbonate (-3.4 vs. -1 mmol/L), sleepiness, and some HRQOL assessments and PSG parameters. Healthcare utilization tended to be lower in the NIV group.
Masa JF et al. Thorax. 2016 Oct;71(10):899-906.

☐

Noninvasive ventilation improves inflammatory and cardiovascular biomarkers in patients with stable hypercapnic COPD. Blood samples drawn from 20 COPD patients before and after 3 months of noninvasive positive pressure ventilation showed significant improvements in $PaCO_2$ during nighttime ventilation and daytime spontaneous breathing, and BNP. Reduction in $PaCO_2$ was associated with a decrease in BNP. Slightly lower levels of IL-10 were also seen.
Dreher M et al. Respir Med. 2015 Oct;109(10):1300-4.

☐

Chronic O_2 therapy has varying effects in different patients with OHS. This is a *post hoc* analysis of an earlier RCT that randomly assigned 302 patients with OHS to NIV, CPAP or lifestyle modification. After 2 months of follow-up, supplemental O_2 increased metabolic alkalosis and decreased AHI in the lifestyle modification group, increased the frequency of morning confusion in the CPAP group, and possibly reduced systolic BP in the NIV group.
Masa JF et al. J Clin Sleep Med. 2016 Oct 15;12(10):1379-1388.

☐
Loudness of snoring increases in proportion to the severity of OSA.
Home sleep testing and snoring loudness were evaluated in 404 patients.
Mean AHI was 16.5 ± 15.3. The AHI correlated with both mean snoring
intensity and percent sleep time with snoring intensity greater than 50
dB. Mean snoring loudness in moderate and severe OSA were 47.7 ± 5.0
and 50.5 ± 5.6 dB, respectively.
Kim JW et al. Clin Exp Otorhinolaryngol. 2015 Dec;8(4):376-380.

☐
**Patients with severe OSA have higher maximal snoring sound frequency
and louder snoring sound intensity.** This study investigated the
relationship between OSA severity and snoring sounds in 103 snoring
subjects. Snoring sounds were recorded and analyzed for maximal
frequency and average snoring sound intensity. Both snoring parameters
correlated with AHI, REM AHI, OSA severity, mean SaO_2 and SaO_2min.
Acar M et al. Ann Otol Rhinol Laryngol. 2016 Jan;125(1):31-6.

☐
Snoring intensity is not affected by AHI and is similar in both genders.
Analysis of snoring characteristics was conducted on 121 subjects using
noncontact ambient microphone during PSG. Snoring index (events per
hour) was higher for men and in N3 sleep compared to N2 and REM
sleep.
Levartovsky A et al. J Clin Sleep Med. 2015 Oct 22.

☐
**There is an association between snoring intensity and daytime
sleepiness in patients without OSA.** Polysomnography was used to
identify 307 simple snorers (AHI < 5) in this prospective cohort study.
Each subject was tested for snoring intensity and sleepiness (ESS
scores ≥ 11). Snoring intensity was similar in both genders, but men were
sleepier than women. Sleepiness (ESS scores) and maximal snoring
intensities were positively correlated.
Kalchiem-Dekel O et al. Laryngoscope. 2016 Feb 10.

☐

Adverse events associated with self-reported snoring include poor sleep patterns, CAD and depression. Analysis of the Behavioral Risk Factor Surveillance System showed that 52.8% of 8,137,604 respondents snored. Snoring was associated with less sleep time, more days with "lack of sleep" or with "unintentional falling asleep", and greater likelihood of falling asleep while driving. Snoring did not increase the risk for strokes.
Bhattacharyya N. Laryngoscope. 2015 Oct;125(10):2413-6.

☐

Snoring is independently associated with LVH. This is a cross-sectional study of 10,139 participants who answered a structured questionnaire on snoring status and intensity. Prevalence of LVH increased with snoring intensity – 10.3% (low snoring intensity), 13.1% (normal intensity), 14.7% (strong intensity), and 16.7% (very strong intensity).
Zhang N et al. BMC Cardiovasc Disord. 2016 Jan 15;16(1):15.

☐

Snoring is an independent risk factor for dyslipidemia and metabolic syndrome in adolescents and young adults. Data from the 2nd Chilean Health Survey included 2,147 subjects (mean age 27.9 ± 7.6 years). Snoring, short sleep duration and metabolic syndrome were present in 43.5, 25% and 19.5% of the subjects, respectively. In an adjusted regression model, odds of metabolic syndrome and elevated cholesterol, but not HTN, were significantly higher among snoring subjects.
Brockmann PE et al. Int J Obes (Lond). 2016 Aug 1.

☐

Snoring increases local oxidative stress in the airways of patients with OSA. In a prospective observational case-control study, researchers measured 8-isoprostane (8-IPN) in exhaled breath condensate prior to CPAP treatment and again after 4 months in 20 patients with OSA and in 10 controls. The only significant predictor of 8-IPN on multivariate analysis was snoring. Levels of 8-IPN decreased after nasal CPAP therapy.
Fernandez Alvarez R et al. Lung. 2016 Jun;194(3):469-73.

☐

Performance of different sensors used to measure snoring varies. In 10 subjects who reported habitual snoring, a chest microphone detected more snore events than an overhead audio, piezoelectric sensor or nasal pressure transducer (cannula), and was able to pick up snore events with lower volume and higher frequency.

Arnardottir ES et al. J Sleep Res. 2015 Nov 9.